Signore, Ascolta!

(Sir, Listen!)

My Journey
with
Brain Cancer

by
Zhila Kashaninia

CCB Publishing
British Columbia, Canada

Signore, Ascolta! My Journey with Brain Cancer

Copyright ©2019 by Zhila Kashaninia
ISBN-13   978-1-77143-405-8
First Edition

Library and Archives Canada Cataloguing in Publication
Title: Sir, listen! = Signore, ascolta! : my journey with brain cancer
/ by Zhila Kashaninia.
Other titles: Signore, ascolta!
Names: Kashaninia, Zhila, 1963- author.
Description: First edition.
Identifiers: Canadiana (print) 20190216786 | Canadiana (ebook) 20190216808 |
ISBN 9781771434058 (softcover) | ISBN 9781771434065 (PDF)
Subjects: LCSH: Kashaninia, Zhila, 1963-—Health. |
LCSH: Brain—Cancer—Patients—British Columbia—Biography. |
LCSH: Brain—Tumors—Patients—British Columbia—Biography. |
LCSH: Brain—Surgery—Patients—California—Los Angeles—Biography. |
LCSH: Medical tourism—United States. | LCGFT: Autobiographies.
Classification: LCC RC280.B7 K37 2019 | DDC 362.19699/4810092—dc23

Front & back cover artwork credit: Photos of Zhila Kashaninia by
Heather Stone, Tulle and Tweed Photography, Victoria, BC, Canada
Website: https://tulleandtweedphotography.com

Disclaimer: SEE YOUR PHYSICIAN. The information in this book is not
intended to replace that of your physician and does not constitute medical advice.
Do not use this book in place of proper medical care. Readers are advised to seek
professional medical assistance in the event that they are suffering from any
medical problem. All health questions concerning yourself or anyone else, must
initially be addressed by your doctor or physician.

Extreme care has been taken by the author to ensure that all information
presented in this book is accurate and up to date at the time of publishing.
Neither the author nor the publisher can be held responsible for any errors or
omissions. Additionally, neither is any liability assumed for damages resulting
from the use of the information contained herein.

Publisher: CCB Publishing
               British Columbia, Canada
               www.ccbpublishing.com

Dedicated to Dr. Daniel F. Kelly

Whose brilliance, kindness, and
generosity are unparalleled

"I wish I could show you...
the astonishing light of your being."

~Hafez (1315-1390)

Contents

The Day Before...

Listening to Montserrat Caballé singing *Signore, ascolta* while driving to teach a course on *Voices in Opera* at the university, I think to myself: I have spent 25 years exploring my own voice and teaching students about the importance of breath and how they can gain freedom in their bodies with yoga to develop their voices with correct technique, and I am still amazed at how this lady is able to sing the B flat at the end with such delicate pianissimo and then gradually crescendo and end with so much power. I wonder what Puccini's reaction would have been if he had heard Caballé while composing his *Turandot?* My colleagues and I still listen with absolute wonder and awe!

Still immersed in thoughts about the human voice and how it is able to transport us to places we have never been but want to go, I arrive at the university. I park my car and head to the classroom with my laptop in one hand and files in the other. First, I set up, attaching the laptop to the projector, checking the sound, and feeling the usual butterflies and anxious energy. I remember a friend once told me, *"When you stop feeling the butterflies, that's the time to quit teaching!"*

Students begin to arrive. I greet everyone and begin the class by talking about the human voice: "Our focus in this course is opera singers—voices that are trained to sing without a microphone in large opera houses of around 1,200 seats in Europe to nearly 4,000 seats at the Metropolitan Opera in New York. In order to be able to do that and have a lasting career, one must rely on excellent breathing technique."

After briefly talking about the anatomy and physiology of the voice, I continue: "Men and women have different vocal folds. Adult males have voices that are usually lower-pitched and have larger vocal folds. The male vocal folds are between 17.5 mm and 25 mm in length. The female vocal folds are between 12.5 mm and 17.5 mm in length. It is important to remember that no two voices are alike, not only because of the size and shape of the vocal folds, but also because of the size and shape of the person's body."

I glance around the room and as I talk so passionately about the subject, I have everyone's attention. I continue with the classification of women's voices: sopranos, mezzo sopranos, and contraltos.

"Tonight, we will focus on sopranos. I will write the main types of sopranos on the board for you. We go from the highest and the lightest and end with the richest and most dramatic: coloratura, soubrette, lyric, spinto, and dramatic."

I patiently go through the classifications and play the best examples in my collection. I look at my audience and the level of astonishment and excitement is mutual. Truly, when I listen to these singers, it is as if I am listening to them for the first time.

Before I know it, I only have a few minutes left. I ask them if they would mind staying for five more minutes to listen to one of my favourite Wagnerian singers: Jessye Norman. Everyone agrees to stay. As the song ends, we are officially ten minutes over, but no one has left the classroom! This is a clear indication that things went well in the first class. I express my thanks to the students for staying and say that I will see them next week.

People gather their belongings and as they leave the room, they smile and say thank you. I slowly gather my things. As I leave the building, I feel the warm air on my skin reminding me of the change of season, but I am still in the world of beautiful singers.

I start the car and Caballé is finishing the aria. I listen to her beautiful ending and decide to play it again. My drive home from the university is 15 minutes, which means I get to listen to her at least two more times!

The Day That Changed My Life

It was 6:30 a.m., and the sun was peeking through the clouds. I slowly opened my eyes. Although staying under the warm covers was very inviting, I convinced myself that a brisk walk would make me feel better. I had so much planned for the day: a meeting with the coordinator at the university about courses for next year, signing up for a yoga therapy workshop, meeting a friend to help her with her résumé, and working on my course proposals for next year.

I dressed and walked outside. The touch of the cool morning air on my face proved that I had made the right decision. As I walked, I thought about life, my courses, and where I needed to take my interests in music and yoga. My proposal on the strong connection between yoga and singing had been accepted at an international conference in Stockholm, Sweden—now the sky was the limit! I was still swimming deeply in my thoughts and possibilities as I walked back to my apartment. I took my jacket off as usual and was heading towards the kitchen to make breakfast when all of a sudden I felt an intense heat around my head. The room was spinning. I took a step but my knees buckled and I fell to the carpeted floor.

The next thing I remembered was opening my eyes and trying to sit up. I thought for a moment about what had taken place and even though I felt well enough, I decided to call 911.

I then called my sister Mina, who lived about five minutes away. Although we are nine years apart, we are very close and happen to be best friends. After I told her what happened, she said she would be over as soon as possible; as it turned out, she arrived right before the ambulance. The paramedics examined me and determined that although my vital signs were normal, I should go to the hospital to be examined. They loaded me into the ambulance and drove to the hospital.

When I arrived at the hospital, I was brought into a private space in the emergency room with curtains drawn and was asked to take everything off, put it all in a bag, and put on the blue hospital gown. I was also fitted with a white plastic bracelet that identifies you as a patient. While lying there, I tried to say something to Mina; all of a sudden, the words would not come out. I could feel my head moving from side to side and could also see the frightened look on Mina's face.

A nurse and doctor came in. I could hear a mixture of sounds—words, movements— and could sense a feeling of urgency. "She is having a seizure…quick!" I could feel pressure on my right arm as an IV pumped anti-seizure medication into my body.

I felt reasonably well after a few minutes. The doctor ordered a CT scan of my brain, which showed a mass. The next step was an MRI. I remembered being told in the conservatory as a student that I had exceptional hearing. While this is very beneficial for a singer and a musician, it puts you at a disadvantage when having an MRI, as every little sound is magnified tenfold.

After the MRI, I was brought back to the room in a wheelchair. Mina had gone to get us coffee. The attending doctor came in and very casually said, "You have a brain tumor. We have set you up with a neurosurgeon to see what he recommends." Shortly after, he left the room. I looked at the white ceiling, contemplating how, in a matter of minutes, my life was so dramatically changed and all my hopes and dreams were shattered. What was going to happen to me? At this moment, all the odds were against me.

I was released from the hospital the next day. As I left the room, I looked at the other patients lying in their beds and wondered whether their stories were as dramatic and complicated as mine. Mina interrupted my thoughts and reminded me that we had to fill a prescription before going home. Even hearing these words was foreign to me. I had never been on any medication before and had lived a healthy life—no alcohol or tobacco use, regular exercise, and a vegetarian diet. How could something like this ever happen to someone like me?

Initial Diagnosis

Inoperable tumor

Time stood still. I remembered Salvador Dali's painting, *The Persistence of Memory*, which he described as clocks losing their power in a dream world, yet this was not a dream to me, and time had so much power over me. It was as if all of a sudden someone had pushed the "pause" button on my life. I cancelled all my music and yoga classes and my meetings and was now focused on reading about my illness. And with all the negative prognoses about "brain tumors", it was hard to be positive and hopeful. The week between my initial release from the hospital and seeing the neurosurgeon seemed more like a month or perhaps even a year.

The day finally arrived to see the neurosurgeon, and I found myself with Mina in his office. He arrived and showed me the MRI of my brain with the tumor. I looked at it in disbelief. Was this really mine? I wanted to escape but the reality was staring me in the face. The doctor said that this was an inoperable tumor, and the best course of action was to have a biopsy to determine what kind of tumor it was, so that it could be treated accordingly.

He also said that there was a 10 percent risk of paralysis on my right side with doing the biopsy. The room went quiet for a moment, and that moment seemed like an eternity. I looked at Mina and we both agreed that the biopsy was my best option even with the risk of paralysis. The surgeon seemed so indifferent. He said that he only performed biopsies on certain days and that I would receive a call once I was scheduled. He then casually got up, closed my file and left the room. I remembered reading about the meaning of the word patient: One who endures, tolerates suffering without becoming annoyed or anxious; indeed, this now was me in every sense of the word.

The Uneasy Week Before the Biopsy

The days continued to pass very slowly. Mina and I decided to tell our other sisters and their families. This unenviable task was left to her, and the number of phone calls and emails that she had to answer was staggering. However, she shielded me from them with such mastery and grace.

We decided to go to Vancouver to see one of my other sisters and her family. Somehow, this weekend visit was not the same as usual, even though everyone tried to make it extra special, with unusual treats and out-of-the-ordinary movies and entertainment. The dark cloud of uncertainty and my almost certain mortality were hanging over us.

On many nights between the initial diagnosis and the day of the biopsy, I was unable to sleep, so I was often up in the early hours of the morning. I tried to read, but even when I opened the most intriguing book and read a sentence or two, my eyes would fall on a blank space on the page and my mind would wander off to the inevitable.

The Epiphany

One early morning two days before the biopsy, I got up and a new thought suddenly came to me. I said to myself, "I have decided to go through the process of biopsy and further treatment and now I have the choice to go through it with fear or to take a more peaceful approach." I remembered the work of Dr. Masaru Emoto (*The Hidden Messages in Water*), where he demonstrated how molecules of water change when given positive and negative thoughts. Dr. Emoto said that if we can see the result of this experiment with glasses of water, the same could be true for our bodies, which comprise over 70 percent water.[1]

What would be the result for me if I approached this situation with fear instead of hope? What would it be like if I replaced fear with peace and hope? I decided to change my way of thinking. Yes, I have a brain tumor but I am not the brain tumor. I am still the person with the same passions, interests, values, and experiences that have made me who I am. As I wrote all these new

---

[1] Masaru Emoto, *The Hidden Messages in Water* (New York: Atria Books, 2005).

thoughts in my journal, I felt surrounded by hope and a sense of strength and felt that now I had what I needed for this challenging journey of mine.

The Day of the Biopsy

I was told to arrive at the hospital at 6:00 a.m. Mina and I took a taxi to be on time. As the taxi passed through the streets, I enjoyed the early morning scenery, the lights, and colours. We arrived at the hospital and had to wait in a room full of people who were also having surgery that day. As I walked up to the desk, the nurse had stepped away and a young man was there waiting. He kindly told us that he was just there to ask a question about his wife and that the nurse would return shortly.

After the nurse was done with our registration and paperwork, we were sent to wait in the next room, and I recognized the young man who was now sitting beside his wife and their young daughter. It appeared that his wife was pregnant and had major complications, since it didn't look like she was ready to give birth yet. She was very calm despite being in pain and was speaking about her situation to the nurse. Her face showed the pain, and her husband was so worried and so attentive to her. Shortly after, the door opened and the young woman was called. She got up and said goodbye to her husband and daughter. Her daughter felt the urgency of the situation and began crying and screaming, "Mommy!"

The mother looked at her daughter, put her hand on her daughter's face, and calmly said, "Remember, Mommy loves you." She then had a tender exchange with her husband and left the room.

I was swimming in my thoughts about this couple and was sending them hope and healing thoughts when I heard my name being called. I was given the familiar blue gown and plastic bag and was given instructions to prepare. Mina was told that she could stay with me until they took me to the operating room. The nurse came in and attached an IV of antibiotics to my arm. She also told us all the things that could possibly go wrong with the biopsy and then turned to Mina and said, "Are you ok?" What a question to ask at such a time!

Soon after, another nurse came in and said to Mina that she was going to take me to the "Theatre", which apparently was the place where they take all the patients before surgery. Mina and I embraced and I told her with a smile that I would see her soon. I didn't have my contact lenses on, so as the nurse took me through the empty hallways, all the coloured lines on the white walls turned into the most intriguing abstract paintings. I enjoyed this display of colour and imagination that momentarily took me to another world.

We soon arrived at the Theatre—quite a different theatre than the ones I was used to in my world. Why do they refer to this place as the Theatre? I tried so desperately to find similarities, something to take me back to the past experiences of performing—backstage in the dark, the nervous energy, performers hugging and wishing each other well, the excitement, going over the fine details, hearing the orchestra tuning. No, there were definitely no similarities.

The Theatre was a large, dark room with patients lined up to be taken to surgery. There was no excitement or creativity, and there was a different kind of nervous energy. I decided to try and amuse myself in an effort to take my mind off of what was going to happen to me. I became interested in the scenery, the lights, and the trivial conversations between the surgeons and nurses. I noticed every little thing, even the sterile smell of the room and the unpleasant taste of the antibiotics at the back of my throat.

The surgeon came into the room, took a look at me, and gave me a formal greeting. The assistant surgeon was much more personable. He had an accent, and when I asked him about it, he said that he was from Georgia, a small country in Eastern Europe very close to Iran. I replied that I was familiar with his home country and that a few famous opera singers came from there. He gave me a surprised look, perhaps thinking to himself, "Does this woman know what she is in for?" I don't think he knew my state of mind and what I had promised myself.

Soon after he left, two men came and took me into the operating room. There were large computer screens with four people setting them up. The two men brought the bed close to the centre of the room and asked me to slide to the operating bed, which was very hard and cold. The anaesthesiologist had a mask in his hand and told me to take a few deep breaths while he put the mask on my face. He said that when I woke up, I would be in the recovery room.

Recovery Room and the
First Night After the Biopsy

I opened my eyes and I was shivering. I could feel my teeth chattering, and when one of the nurses came to check on me she said, "This woman is freezing!" I was soon covered with three warm blankets, which brought some comfort. I could hardly move my head, but I realized that Mina was waiting and needed to know that I was okay. I knew the neurosurgeon was going to call her but I didn't know when this would happen. As hard as it was to move my head, I looked around. I soon saw a nurse sitting and watching me, and also saw a phone very close by. I looked at the nurse from the corner of my left eye, trying to hold my head as still as I possibly could to avoid the excruciating pain. I pleaded with her to call my sister; miraculously, I remembered Mina's cell phone number and gave it to her. The nurse repeated a couple of times that the neurosurgeon would get in touch with the family, but she knew that I wasn't going to give up easily and so she decided to call Mina. Once I heard the conversation and knew that she was talking to Mina, I breathed a sigh of relief. Soon after, the neurosurgeon came and asked me to move my right hand and leg. After seeing that I could, he left without saying a word.

I was soon brought to the neuroscience ward and placed in a room with another patient. I could see Mina and another friend in the room but I felt so weak that I wasn't able to acknowledge them. Mina tried to take my journal and book out of a plastic bag and put them next to me on the side table; however, even the gentle sound of a plastic bag rustling sounded like the harshest thunderstorm to me. I asked her with the few words I could find to stop, and she did so very quickly. The room was kept dark and I soon understood why: every speck of light seemed so harsh to my eyes so I tried to keep them closed.

Mina was soon told to leave as visiting hours were over. I tried to breathe deeply and just meditate. A young nurse came and held my hand. Before she left the room, she said, "Call me if you need anything, even a hug!" I contemplated her kindness for a moment and gently nodded.

The minutes seemed like hours. The nurse's aide came to see if I needed pain medication, and when I asked what type of pain medication they were giving me, she replied that it was morphine. It was interesting going from not even taking a Tylenol to having heavy doses of morphine every two hours, but with the kind of pain I was experiencing, the choice was clear.

My forced tranquility came to an abrupt end when I heard a scream from another room, "Help me!" At first, I thought that perhaps this person was in the same shape or worse off than me, and then I heard that he had a mental illness. The staff left him, thinking that he would soon get tired and quiet down. Instead, he became so desperate that he found a metal utensil and began hitting the side of the bed with it. The sound of metal on metal sent me over the edge. I asked for the kind young nurse, and when she came in, I was hysterically crying. I pleaded with her to move me to another room. She held me and promised that she would do whatever she could for me. She left, and soon returned with another nurse who was hesitant to help. The young nurse insisted that, under the circumstances, they had to try. She then told me that generally, the job of moving patients was left to porters who knew how to navigate the hallways with hospital beds; however, that would take time, so she decided to do it herself with the help of the other nurse.

They brought me to a room down the hall, which had three other women in it. At first, it seemed quiet but that didn't last long. I soon learned about my roommates: The woman next to me had had a stroke, and as a result, her blood pressure and pulse were very low. She was constantly vomiting, but was too weak to get up. The woman in front of her, an international student, had a spinal cord infection and was barely hanging on to life. The woman in front of me looked in the best shape of us all; however, I soon learned that she had had a massive stroke, which caused her to lose her memory almost completely—the only thing she could remember was her name.

Because this was the neuroscience ward, the main doors were locked and visiting hours were limited. The lights were turned off at 9:00 p.m. Given that I had received so much morphine, I hoped to get some sleep, but that was not going to happen. The woman in front of me started to talk to herself. When I called the nurse, she explained that this had happened before and should stop momentarily. She did assure me that if it continued, she would move the woman's bed to the hallway. Luckily, the woman's talking stopped within an hour. I breathed a sigh of relief, but it was short-lived. Soon after, the international student asked to go to the bathroom; upon her return, she had a massive seizure and the doctor and all the nurses on the floor were called in to help her. It took the team some time to manage the situation. Meanwhile, I needed more morphine, as my incision began to really hurt again.

I knew it was the early hours of the morning, so I tried to close my eyes and meditate in the hope of getting some sleep. My meditation was soon interrupted when the heart monitor of the woman next to me started to beep. I pushed the call button for the nurse, who finally came in and fixed the problem. I looked out the window and it was still dark. Wishing for some peace and quiet and uninterrupted rest, I closed my eyes for whatever was left of the night.

The Second Day After the Biopsy

New possibility and an odd encounter

The morning came, and although I didn't get much sleep the night before, I did feel better. I felt encouraged that my pain was relatively better and my speech was much stronger. In addition, I was now receiving morphine injections every six hours instead of every two. I was also able to order breakfast but only managed to eat a banana. For some reason, I was repulsed by the odour of anything cooked.

I noticed a sign on the wall that said visiting hours started at 11:00 a.m. I longed to see a familiar face, someone from my world, but they were quite strict in this ward and I knew that Mina would be here if she could. I looked around and decided to write in my journal. As I began to write, I noticed that my handwriting was the same as before the biopsy and that I could still express my feelings effortlessly. I felt encouraged with every stroke; in an instant, my thoughts were magically translated from my brain to my hand and onto paper. This small—or enormous—act that happened instantly every day for people suddenly seemed incredible to me. My thoughts soon shifted to a fascination with the human body and how it is able to cope with all that we do to it, including abusing it with alcohol, drugs, tobacco, and processed food. In my case, I had caused my body much stress balancing a demanding job with the responsibility of taking care of an elderly family member, which meant at times working 70-hour weeks. The picture was becoming very clear. I was convinced that this experience was going to change my life and teach me the wisdom that I needed for the next chapter of my life.

I was looking out my window, contemplating, when Mina suddenly came in. It was only 8:30 a.m., so I asked her how she was able to come before visiting hours. She said, with a twinkle in her eye, that she had managed to sneak in. She wanted to bring me some fresh fruit and quinoa (my favourite food), but more than that, she was anxious to tell me about the possibility of getting a second opinion from a prominent neurosurgeon in Los Angeles.

The story began when we told our family that my neurosurgeon here had said that my tumor was inoperable. When she heard that, our sister Sheila in San Diego decided to contact her close friend, Jaleh, who was the director of surgical services at the Pacific Neuroscience Institute in Los Angeles. Jaleh said that if we sent a copy of the MRI cd to her, she could get one of their top neurosurgeons to look at it and give us his opinion. The thought of going to the U.S. for surgery and treatment seemed so foreign to me, but I was intrigued to find out if the neurosurgeon in Los Angeles would concur with the neurosurgeon here. I felt in my heart that I should pursue this new possibility.

Mina and I were discussing the easiest way to obtain a copy of the cd when a nurse came in to check my blood pressure. She was surprised to see Mina, and in a scolding tone, informed Mina that visiting hours did not begin until 11:00 a.m. She then asked her to leave. Mina gently pleaded with her to stay, saying that she would be very quiet. The nurse interrupted her and said in no uncertain terms that rules should be respected, because what it would be like if everyone did the same? While this was not what we wanted to hear, under the circumstances we decided that Mina should leave. With the nurse standing by, Mina left, but not before telling me that she would be back at 11:00 a.m. sharp.

On my own again, I thought about what I had heard from Mina about the second opinion. I asked one of the nurses about the quickest way to obtain a cd of my MRI. She said that if I were to ask for it, it would take 40 days, but if the neurosurgeon ordered it, it would take just two days. So my only chance of getting the MRI cd quickly would be through the neurosurgeon who had performed the biopsy, the same man who seemed to regard me only as one of the many cases that he handled every day.

At that very moment, the neurosurgeon came into the room and said casually, "Hi, how are you doing?" I just said that I was fine but wanted to say so much more. He examined my incision and told me that everything looked good, so I would be released from the hospital the next day. He also mentioned that the biopsy results would come in a week and he would let me know as soon as he received them. I thought this was the perfect moment to ask him about the MRI cd. I told him that I had an opportunity to get a second opinion from the Pacific Neuroscience Institute in Los Angeles, and asked if he could request a copy of the MRI cd for me. To my surprise, he became angry, raised his voice and said in a tone of protest, "I don't understand, you don't even have a first opinion and you want a second opinion, and from CALIFORNIA of all places???"

I felt vulnerable and defeated but I gathered every ounce of strength I could find and calmly responded, "You know, this has just come to me without even looking for it so wouldn't it be to my benefit to just see what they would say?"

He looked away and left the room without saying a word. I didn't know what to think, but I knew in my heart that I should pursue this possibility. While I was busy thinking about strategies, the neurosurgeon walked back in the room to inform me that I was wrong in saying that it would take 40 days to get the MRI cd; in fact, he said, it would only take two days. Without waiting for me to respond, he left the room. I thought to myself, how could I be wrong about something like this? In the past, I was known among family and friends for having a great memory. Could that all be in the past? Was I facing a new world of not remembering and forgetting something so important? I realized that what was important now was to obtain this cd the fastest way possible, so I slowly walked over to the nurses' station and found the kind young nurse that I had met after my biopsy. She asked me what I was doing out of bed. I responded that I wanted to order a copy of my MRI cd. She informed me that the neurosurgeon had already requested it for me. I thanked her and slowly headed back to the room. I was surprised that the neurosurgeon had done this after the way he talked to me. I was grateful and I thanked him, in my mind, even though he never gave me the opportunity to do so in person.

As I slowly walked back to my room, I looked at the patients in the adjacent rooms who were like me—not well, vulnerable, dependant, and at the mercy of powerful individuals with letters beside their names and stethoscopes around their necks who made crucial decisions on our behalf. Did they know that with a "yes" or "no" and the stroke of a pen on paper, they held our fate in their hands, of just existing as opposed to fully participating in this world?

At 11:00, Mina returned with coffee. I was happy to see her and told her the story. She looked at me in disbelief but said that the result was positive and that was all that was important. Seeing positive results despite the agonies of achieving them was a special quality in Mina that I always appreciated.

That afternoon, a couple of friends came for a visit. It was so nice to see them and to hear from them that I looked good, despite having gone through a major biopsy and having multiple stitches on my head. It was nice to have contact with the outside world, being reassured that life still existed outside the hospital and was not out of reach for me.

Mina stayed with me until 6:00 p.m., when I asked her to leave. She wanted to make sure that I was ok, and once I convinced her, she left. I was looking forward to a night of rest. Things were more stable with the other patients in the room compared to the previous night. So I read a few pages of my book and soon felt tired and fell asleep.

Dark Delusions

I was suddenly awakened by the sound of the call button of the woman next to me. When I opened my eyes, I had the most frightening experience. I looked around the room and everything was distorted. The window was on the floor, my feet were on the ceiling and my head was on the floor. I closed my eyes, thinking that this was just a bad dream. I slowly opened them and everything was still distorted. What is happening to my mind, I thought. I didn't have an answer. I quickly sat up and somehow everything instantly returned to normal. However, when I tried to lie down again, I quickly lost perspective of everything again. At this point, my heart was beating rapidly so I pushed the call button with no hesitation. When the nurse came, I told her what was happening and she took my blood pressure: it was 165 over 85. I thought for sure that she would write in my chart that I should undergo another close evaluation before being released from the hospital the next day. What she said was not even close to what I was thinking. "I think you should go home tomorrow. I think that would be so much better for you." And she offered me the option of sitting in the hallway with a warm blanket.

I graciously accepted, picked up my journal and my pen and followed her to the hallway.

There was a little light and a semi-comfortable chair, so I sat and started to madly write. I wrote about anything and everything. I was grateful that I was still able to do this task that I once took for granted. However, I also felt that this was the beginning of the end. Tears fell down my face for the first time since this ordeal began. I was going down a dark path, thinking about what I had lost. I thought about what would come next. Whatever this tumor was, perhaps the delusions were part of it. I couldn't help but mourn the eventual loss of my dreams, my ambitions, my music, and most importantly, my ability to learn, analyze, and process concepts.

The reality of my condition was now staring me in the face. I had to find more courage and become stronger. All the tears in the world would not resolve anything and I could never go back to where I was before. I needed to hang on to something positive, something beautiful that I could feel at this very moment. And yes, I found Caballé's *Signore, ascolta* again. I could hear her singing so clearly in my mind. I could hear how beautifully she navigated to the high B flat. I played that piece over and over in my head and saw myself talking about it so enthusiastically in my class. All of a sudden, I felt lighter and at peace. I thought of the beautiful life I led and all the amazing experiences I had. I thought to myself that wherever this journey was taking me, I would take it step by step. And I would never again ask why me, but *why not me*.

I looked at the clock and it was 4:25 a.m. Three hours had passed and it felt like an eternity. I was tired but was afraid to lie down and experience the dark delusions again, so I continued to sit and listen to the conversation of the young nurses. Most of their discussion was about how difficult night shift can be on their families. Then, one of them started to talk about the interesting mysteries of working nights. She talked about the haunted parts of the hospital, where people had seen ghosts, and how one should never go to these places alone. I listened to these stories and wondered to myself, would seeing ghosts be worse than having an unknown brain tumor, multiple stitches on the scalp, delusions, and all the unknown problems to come? I smiled, rested my head back on the chair and closed my eyes.

Hospital Release After the Biopsy

Subtle uncomfortable changes

It was shortly after 6:00 a.m. I had not heard anything about not being released from the hospital, so I began to get dressed and packed to go home. I went to the bathroom and looked at myself in the mirror. My pale face with the dark circles under my eyes portrayed a clear picture of what had taken place in the last two days. My hair was clearly shaved 2 inches in the middle and also on the left side in order to do the biopsy. I could see a number of metal stitches from the hairline to the middle of my head. The nurse had given me a small comb but the thought of trying to comb my hair even lightly felt impossible, so I decided to not even try it. I said to myself that there is no point in fighting reality. I felt reasonably well and that was all that was important at the moment.

I wanted to go out for a walk but I was told that I had to stay on the same floor. I thought it was better to walk rather than just sit and wait, so I walked the hallway a couple of times, looking for inspirations, smiles, perhaps someone going home. But I could not find anything so I came back to my room. I sat on the bed and started to write. As the words appeared on the page, I was grateful that I still had the ability to formulate sentences and transfer them to the page so easily. I was also grateful to have pen and paper, as it brought me joy just to write about everything that I observed.

Mina soon came with coffee and treats. She was surprised to see me dressed and ready to go. We thought that we should stop at the nurse's station and ask when we could expect to receive the MRI cd. The nurse told us that if we waited for a couple of hours, it would be delivered to us. We were told that we could wait in a small room reserved for patients and their families.

Mina and I decided to amuse ourselves with my music files on my laptop. I showed her the great singers of the past and present, and she played along with my overabundance of enthusiasm. We listened to the greats—Montserrat Caballé, Maria Callas, Tito Gobbi, Léopold Simoneau, Leontyne Price, Jessye Norman, to name a few—and truly experienced the idea that time was a relative concept. Before we knew it, a nurse came into the room and handed us the MRI cd. I went to the desk and found the kind young nurse I had met on the day of the biopsy. I gave her a hug and thanked her for her kindness. She was overjoyed that I was being released.

Home After the Biopsy

*How I respond to my diagnosis
is completely up to me!*

The first night in my apartment, I woke up at 3:45 a.m. At first, I was afraid to open my eyes, but when did, I noticed that everything was where it was supposed to be, and there was no loss of perspective. I breathed a sigh of relief. The familiar environment of home seemed very comforting and welcoming. There was a sliver of light entering from the window that hinted at the coming of dawn. I began to write in my journal. This whole experience seemed surreal, as if I was outside of my body watching it happen.

I was sent home with a medication (dexamethasone) to reduce the inflammation of the brain after the biopsy, added to the anti-seizure medication that I had been taking for the last month. Although weight gain was listed as one of the side effects of dexamethasone, for me it was the complete opposite—I had almost no appetite. Even my favourite foods tasted like I was chewing on wood. I started to lose weight and had horrifying thoughts of what could happen with chemotherapy and radiation.

Mina decided to stay with me for the time being. She did all the housework and cooking, accompanied me to all the appointments, and provided so much emotional support. I think I always knew how caring she was but the extent of it now was beyond imagination, and now I needed her help more than ever. Although I was relatively well, I could not stand longer than a few minutes. I would forget a few words here and there and sometimes when Mina said something, I couldn't quite grasp the meaning of it. Mina was so patient with me, and made nothing out of my lapses. But I knew that something was not quite right, as I often found that my mind was ahead of my speaking ability. Not being able to say the words that my brain had already signalled sent my heart racing and left me out of breath. It was frightening at first but I found a way of managing it. With the first symptom, I slowed down, sat, and breathed deeply with my eyes closed. After a few minutes, all would be well.

A few days passed, and I felt strong enough to go out for coffee. Mina left me at home to go to her apartment for a couple of hours before we headed to our favourite café. I had more energy and was able to do some cooking and other light work around the house. I was so happy for the littlest things that I could accomplish. This was the first time I was alone in my home—just me and my thoughts. I listened to Erik Satie's *Gnossienne No. 1*, and despite its melancholy mood, there was a sense of strength and hope in Satie's music that juxtaposed my own situation. I felt that I had to fight and reclaim my life. It was amazing that all the answers were coming to me so clearly. I was learning that no matter what happened, fear only brought negativity and defeat; at every stage, it was up to me to decide what thought process I would bring to my situation.

I needed to get ready to go for coffee. I had to come up with something to cover my head, which was not only shaved in the middle but had these metal stitches from the front of my forehead at the start of the hairline to the middle of my head. It was too hot to wear a hat so I decided to be creative and wrapped a wide, black, cotton belt around my head. I looked at myself in the mirror and was pleased with the result.

Mina arrived and complimented me on my look, and we were soon on our way. When we arrived at the café, I saw one of my colleagues whom I hadn't seen for many years. We talked briefly, and I decided not to mention my illness. He commented so positively on my new "fashion statement." I thanked him and said to myself...*If only he knew.*

Hearing the News of
My Untimely Death

About a week after the biopsy, I went to see my physician, Dr. Davison, to remove my stitches. As he removed the stitches, he informed me that he had just received my pathology report and the result of the biopsy. My tumor was described as a grade II oligodendroglioma. He said that he was not well versed in brain tumors but as far as he knew, it was a rare, malignant tumor for which the life expectancy was anywhere from three to ten years. He concluded that given my age, I was looking at a maximum of five years.

I was numb and wanted to be anywhere but where I was at that moment. Dr. Davison kept talking about appointments with the oncologist and radiologist for chemotherapy and radiation, but I was not listening. I knew Mina would remember everything, and I thought about how difficult this must be for her to hear. I was also physically in pain because one of the stitches being removed started to bleed. I used this as an excuse to go to the bathroom. I looked at myself in the mirror and saw someone whose hopes and dreams no longer remained. What would life represent for me from now until the inevitable? The whole experience seemed surreal. Was this really how it was all going to end?

I came back to the room to get my bag and saw the most compassionate look on Dr. Davison's face. He told me that his door was always open to me and I could come and see him any time. I was touched so much by this kind gesture, because it provided a ray of light in a moment of absolute darkness.

Mina and I walked for more than an hour without saying a word to each other. When we arrived downtown, we decided to go for lunch. During lunch, we talked about the time I had left and what I really wanted to do. Mina calculated the time to be over 1,700 days. I started to think of this experience as a gift. How many people are given the opportunity to know how long they have to live and then really live their life to the fullest? I gathered my thoughts and put things in perspective. So many questions remained: What did I need to do that would be fulfilling for me with the time I had left? What was really important to me? It was surprising what came to my mind. The idea of going on exotic trips and achieving bigger and better things wasn't really part of it. What came to me immediately, and soon became monumentally important, was what was happening to me at that moment: seeing myself with Mina in the restaurant, tasting the food and being truly present in the moment. I was aware of the pattern, texture, and vibrant colours of the tablecloth; the sharp and sweet taste on my tongue of the vinegar and basil in the salad dressing; and the deep scent of cilantro and curry from the table next to us. All of a sudden, I felt how rich and full life can be, by truly sensing what we often consider to be small, insignificant things. I realized that many of us look for so much outside of ourselves all our lives.

As we walked home, the colour of the flowers and the leaves on the trees suddenly became more vibrant. The deep shades of orange, red, yellow, and green all seemed so incredibly intense and magical. I looked up at the sky and saw the beauty of the soft blue sky accompanied by the pure white clouds. Such beautiful harmony was beyond my comprehension. I noticed the wonder of nature around me and all it had to offer; yet, this was all here before. Clearly, I was the one who was changed and I was now able to sense all of this on another level.

Two Neurosurgeons...
Two Conflicting Opinions

Shortly after we returned home, we received a call from the neurosurgeon. He said that the results of the pathology report were back—which we knew already. According to him, the results were great news. He said that the grade II oligodendroglioma was the best type of tumor to have, since it grew very slowly and was very sensitive to chemotherapy and radiation. He advised that he would set up appointments for me to start treatment the following week. When I asked about my life expectancy, he said I was looking at about ten years. I thanked him and hung up the phone. Mina and I embraced and revelled in the joy of me having a few more years now.

Later that day, we sent the pathology report to our sister Sheila to forward to her friend Jaleh in Los Angeles. The quickness of the response and the difference in the opinion of the neurosurgeon in Los Angeles was a surprise to us all. The response was from a prominent neurosurgeon by the name of Dr. Daniel Kelly. His tone was very friendly, and I felt his sincerity even through his few written words. He said that, in no uncertain terms, my best option would be to have surgery to remove as much of the tumor as possible (at least 80 to 90 percent) before chemotherapy and radiation. Dr. Kelly insisted that this approach would give me the longest possible life expectancy.

Receiving all of this information at once was overwhelming. Two experienced neurosurgeons had given me their opinions: one said that the tumor was inoperable, while the other said that it was operable and that my chance of survival was lower if it was not removed.

Mina and I talked to our sister Lila in Vancouver, who suggested that we meet with Dr. Cameron, a neurologist in Vancouver, to get his opinion on the situation. We also decided to try and talk to Dr. Kelly ourselves.

Meanwhile, I thought that I should make an appointment with the neurosurgeon who performed my biopsy to show him Dr. Kelly's opinion. I called his office and mentioned the nature of my call. I said that I had received a second opinion, and I would like to have the neurosurgeon's email in order to forward the opinion to him. His secretary informed me that they were not allowed to share his email with patients. The only possible option was for me to send the email to her so she could forward it to him. She also said that the earliest appointment would be in three weeks. This was frustrating to me, as I wanted to explain the whole situation to give context to the email, but the only option now was to explain the situation to the secretary and hope for the best. I pondered the huge fortress that was being built in front of me.

The next day, Mina and I went to see Dr. Davison, my doctor, to get a referral to see Dr. Cameron, the neurologist in Vancouver. When we mentioned receiving the opinion from the neurosurgeon in Los Angeles, Dr. Davison said right away that Los Angeles was on the cutting edge when it came to brain surgery and was ahead of everyone with the latest technology and surgical techniques. In fact, he said that if he were in my position, he would go there without hesitation. We left the doctor's office with much-needed hope.

Meanwhile, I wanted to learn more about Dr. Kelly. When I saw his profile, I was impressed not only with all his achievements and awards, but also with the two-minute video on the website where he said: "When you are treating patients with brain tumors, it is important to feel that they are like members of your family."

I decided to call his office to see if I could schedule a phone call with him. I asked if I could email Dr. Kelly directly and his secretary was very surprised at my question and gave me his email right away. This informal approach was in contrast to my earlier experience and was quite comforting.

I emailed Dr. Kelly and asked when would be a good time to call him. Within an hour, he responded with a suggestion to talk on Saturday morning at 9:30 a.m. I was overjoyed that he cared enough to arrange to call me on the weekend. I answered yes with no hesitation.

I was up at 4:30 a.m. on Saturday morning after getting only five hours of sleep—a routine that was becoming normal to me. I was particularly anxious as I was expecting the call from Dr. Kelly. The thought of going to Los Angeles to have such major surgery was still surreal to me. I had always advocated for people to have surgery and treatment as close to their homes as possible because I believed that people heal faster in their own environment, and now I was considering having brain surgery in another country! In addition, although the financial cost of the surgery was not staggering, it was still a consideration, since in Canada my surgery would be covered under our publicly funded health care system. I was fortunate to own my apartment, as I could always get a mortgage to pay for the surgery. A few years earlier, I was so proud that I was able to achieve my goal of being mortgage-free by the age of 50. I realized how arbitrary our life plans could be, as now in the face of adversity, disability, and possible mortality, none of this seemed to matter.

Over breakfast, Mina and I couldn't help but talk about what was going to happen. We were both anxious and together wrote all the possible questions we could think of to ask Dr. Kelly. Finally, the much-anticipated call came at exactly 9:30 a.m. A feeling of hope filled every corner of the room. I had to curb my anxious feelings and stay focussed. The pleasant and calm voice of Dr. Kelly was already restoring my confidence. He explained that the type of tumor I had was relatively slow growing, and based on a number of excellent studies of low-grade gliomas, maximal safe surgical removal was the best course of action for long-term survival and for maintaining the best quality of life.

I asked him about the risks of the surgery and things that could possibly go wrong. He responded that with this type of tumor and where it was situated, and given the fact that I didn't have conditions such as diabetes, high-blood pressure, or other comorbidities, there was little possibility of complications. However, Dr. Kelly also said that the surgery would be major—it would take five to six hours. I would be in the hospital for two to three nights after and then would need to stay for another week in Los Angeles for appointments with their neuro-oncologist for further treatment suggestions. He also mentioned that in some cases, people with these types of tumors in this particular location could come out of the surgery with a weaker right side; however, in nearly all cases, the weakness only lasted a few weeks. He also thought that the seizures I had experienced showed that the tumor was clearly causing significant distortion and pressure on the surrounding area due to its close proximity to the motor cortex area in the brain. He felt that the surgery should happen very soon, so we talked about tentatively scheduling it for the second week of July, nearly a month and a half after my initial seizure and diagnosis.

After he calmly answered all my questions, Dr. Kelly said, "If you have any other questions, you have my cell phone number now, so you can call me any time." I compared this approach to the distant approach of the neurosurgeon who did my biopsy and was in total amazement of the difference. I thanked Dr. Kelly and we ended the call.

Later that day, I looked at my cell phone and saw Dr. Kelly's name and phone number and reviewed his last words in my mind: *you can call me any time if you have any questions.* I closed my eyes for a moment and felt the power of those simple yet profound words that meant so much to me.

My Friend Sholeh

Reconnecting with the past

One night a couple of years ago, I embarked on a venture to find a couple of good friends from my youth at school in Iran. I looked for them on Facebook and to my surprise, I found them and sent them friend requests. One of these friends was Sholeh. After Sholeh received my friend request, we decided to have a phone conversation and catch up on nearly 38 years of being away from each other. It was so beautiful to reconnect with her. We talked about our lives: the achievements, the struggles, the trials, and the disappointments. We marvelled at how close we felt to each other even after just one phone call, after being apart for all these years. During our conversation, Sholeh briefly mentioned that among her life struggles, she had had brain surgery. I was very surprised to hear this but felt that I shouldn't pry, so I didn't ask anything more about it.

Now, a couple of years later, I had been diagnosed with a brain tumor myself. I was intrigued to talk to Sholeh about her experience. I thought about it for a few days and finally decided to call her. After talking to her about the nature of my call, she asked about the details of my tumor. I told her what type of tumor I had, and she calmly said that I would be fine and that I needed to find a good neurosurgeon. She said that in her case, she did a lot of research and found an excellent neurosurgeon named Dr. Daniel Kelly. She was about to tell me about him, but I interrupted her to mention my connection to Dr. Kelly and how I was also considering having my surgery in Los Angeles. Sholeh was so surprised and overjoyed to hear this news. She said that I had nothing to worry about and had to trust that I was putting my life in the greatest hands. She also said that she lived about ten minutes from the hospital where the surgery was going to take place and that she would come and visit me. It was such a surreal feeling. I told her that I never imagined us reconnecting like this after all these years. I had had a romantic notion of meeting in a quiet café somewhere and catching up on nearly 40 years of lost time. Once again, the lesson was that life doesn't always present us with experiences wrapped in tidy, clean packages with ribbons around them. An experience so much more important was going to take place, and I was feeling its enormity with every ounce of my being.

Before we said good-bye, Sholeh said, "Just remember you now have another sister in Los Angeles." My eyes filled with tears as I expressed my gratitude to her. I promised to call her as soon as I finalized my plans.

Meeting Dr. Cameron

"So much we don't know"

When my sister Lila had mentioned seeing Dr. Cameron, the neurologist in Vancouver, I hesitated at first, because he was a neurologist, not a neurosurgeon, and I thought that with two conflicting opinions from two neurosurgeons, it might make sense to consult another neurosurgeon. However, Lila had always spoken highly of Dr. Cameron as a caring neurologist and a very special human being, so I welcomed the opportunity to meet with him.

I was given the first appointment of the day, so Lila, Mina and I arrived and sat in the waiting room. While waiting, I noticed the native art displayed on nearly every wall, which to me revealed so much about this doctor even before I got the chance to meet him. It didn't take long before a tall, seasoned gentleman walked out and called my name. Lila, Mina, and I followed him to his office. He asked about my situation and after I told him my story, he paused briefly and then said that it made sense to him to have the surgery, as chemotherapy and radiation would be more effective on a smaller tumor.

He then asked me to accompany him to the other room for further examination. When I sat on the bed, I noticed pictures with rainbows and mentioned that he must really like rainbows. He looked at me intensely with his deep blue eyes and asked me what I did for a living. I replied that I taught singing, opera history, and yoga. He smiled and told me that he himself had come close to death two years ago when a virus attacked his immune system and his organs began to shut down. And then all of a sudden, after a few days he started to feel better. After he was released from the hospital, he thought about retirement but felt the need to stay and take care of his patients. He asked me if my experience of the world around me seemed any different after my diagnosis. I told him about experiencing the real beauty of nature, the intensity of colours in flowers and leaves, as if seeing them for the first time. Without uttering a word, his sincere smile showed his agreement with my experience.

He then told me about Thomas Banyacya, one of the four elders of the Hopi Nation in Arizona who was appointed to reveal traditional Hopi wisdom and truth. These native leaders protested the mining of uranium, which was used to make the atomic bombs that were dropped on Hiroshima and Nagasaki in 1945. Dr. Cameron said that he and his wife often visited Thomas and his wife in Arizona. On one occasion, when Thomas saw him, he told Dr. Cameron that he was a compassionate healer beyond his medical training. Sometime later, after Thomas had passed away, Thomas's wife said that Thomas had asked her to give his bracelet that he wore all the time to Dr. Cameron. Although he was hesitant at first, Dr. Cameron graciously accepted the gift.

My eyes were glued to him as he was telling me this incredible story. I tried so hard not to miss a word or even a gesture of this unusual yet profound encounter. For a moment, I even forgot why I was there and felt like I was in a completely different space and time.

He asked me if I wanted to see the bracelet and seeing my enthusiasm, proceeded to roll up his sleeve, revealing the bracelet. He then took it off and placed it in my hands. On the outside, the bracelet looked quite ordinary—it was silver with three turquoise stones. However, once I held it in my hands, the energy emanating from it was incredible. He said that although he was a scientist, the experiences he had gone through had made him open to ideas that were foreign to him before. He went on to say, "There is so much we don't know."

For a moment, I felt a shiver over my entire body. He looked intensely at me and said, "You realize that you being here is not just about your brain tumor. We were meant to meet each other." He then proceeded to tell me that this illness was going to make me into a much more special and effective teacher and that I would be able to inspire and help so many more people.

I agreed with him and said that I would do this as long as I had the mental capacity to teach and help people. I then told him about my delusions after the biopsy. He smiled and said that what had happened had nothing to do with my tumor; instead, it was an allergic reaction to morphine. He said that I should make sure to tell the neurosurgeon about this allergy as it was bound to happen again. I sighed in relief and was grateful to learn about this explanation for my delusions. He then took his fountain pen out of his pocket and wrote the name Thomas Banyacya on a piece of paper. He gave it to me and told me to read about him. I graciously took the paper and put it in my wallet.

Before we left his office, Dr. Cameron said that he would arrange for me to see a prominent neurosurgeon in Vancouver just to have another opinion. I expressed my gratitude and left. At that moment, it was hard for me to imagine that I was going to be fine; yet, he had added the possibility of hope to an existing feeling deep in my heart. Somehow I knew I would see him again.

Appointment with the Neurosurgeon in Victoria

Sudden change of opinion

The day of our meeting with the neurosurgeon in Victoria to discuss Dr. Kelly's opinion had arrived. Mina and I planned to be in the office early.

When we arrived at the office, the radio was blasting the most obtrusive rock music. I looked around to see if this was also bothering others in the waiting room and I discovered that it was. I tried to get the attention of the receptionists but was unsuccessful. So I took matters into my own hands. I spotted the radio, went over to it, and turned it down to the lowest possible volume. In response, I received a couple of smiles and nods indicating a silent applause for my *action without permission*.

After waiting nearly half an hour, we were instructed by one of the receptionists to go into one of the examination rooms. Later, the neurosurgeon came in and sat down. After a few greetings, I asked him to explain his opinion of the tumor being inoperable given the new opinion from Dr. Kelly. He said in the most intimidating tone, "You are a singer, aren't you? Isn't that important to you? Removing 85 to 90 percent of the tumor brings a high risk of speech problems, since the tumor is very close to your speech area. You may never be able to sing again." Hearing this from him left me confused in more ways than one. First, I didn't remember telling him that I was a singer. Second, it would be foolish of me to want to save my voice in the face of disability and possible death.

As I was gathering my thoughts to respond to him in the most appropriate way, he said, "In the U.S., the approach is to operate on everything. In my opinion, your best options are chemotherapy and radiation. I have set you up with an oncologist and radiologist to get the treatment that is right for you."

I responded with the opinion from Dr. Cameron, that it would make sense to have surgery first to remove as much of the tumor as possible before introducing chemotherapy and radiation, in order to get the best possible result. He looked at my chart and said that he wanted to look at my MRI again. He brought up the picture of my tumor on his computer screen and then casually said, "You know, I can do this too."

Just to be clear, I asked, "You mean you would operate to remove 80 percent of the tumor?"

He responded, "Yes, and I can do it just as the surgeon in Los Angeles suggests."

A feeling of fear and distrust ran through my entire body. I could feel my heartbeat quickening and wanted nothing else but to leave his office and never return. I calmly mentioned that I was also seeking an opinion from a neurosurgeon in Vancouver. He quickly agreed that this was a good idea and suggested that it would be best if I didn't mention Dr. Kelly's opinion to the neurosurgeon in Vancouver, so that I received an unbiased opinion. He again reiterated that he would be happy to accommodate me with the surgery should I wish to have the surgery at home.

Mina and I both thanked him and said we would think about it and let him know. He acted like a true gentleman by opening the door for us and saying a proper farewell. Somehow, it didn't seem sincere to me. When we were out of the office, I asked Mina what she felt in her heart about what we had experienced. Without hesitation, she uttered the words that expressed my own exact sentiments, "We should go to Los Angeles."

The Start of Planning to Go to Los Angeles

Planning to have brain surgery far away from home

After hearing that we had to wait for nearly a month to see the neurosurgeon in Vancouver, we were all convinced that it was a good idea to start planning for Los Angeles. After we received the proposed date for the surgery, we began preparing for this uneasy trip. It was so beautiful and comforting to know that not only Mina (from Victoria) and Lila (from Vancouver) were going to accompany me to Los Angeles but also my sister Roya and her husband Farid from Dallas, Texas, as well as my sister Sheila and her husband Mehdi from San Diego. We decided not to tell my mother and brother, who lived in San Diego, since my brother had had a challenging back surgery and was still in the hospital. Again, this was another lesson that life events don't always happen based on our schedules and often present their own unexpected challenges.

I had never been to Los Angeles and here I was planning to have brain surgery in this city that was completely unknown to me. Now more than ever, I needed courage and trust. Somehow, brain cancer has a way of getting a hold of you and making you forget who you are and what you have accomplished. I had to constantly remind myself that if I forgot, misplaced, or lost something or dropped and broke a plate or glass, it had nothing to do with my malignant brain tumor and it was normal. NORMAL…what a word! All my life, I wanted to be different and now every ounce of my being longed to be associated with the word normal.

I also had to learn to accept all that was being offered to me by family and friends. This wasn't easy for me, as I had been away from my parents and on my own since age fifteen. All my sisters and my brothers-in-law were offering support, each in their own unique way, from cooking my favourite foods, to long, deep telephone conversations, to sending prayers and positive thoughts. I had to learn that human beings are unique and respond in their own way to a challenging illness in someone they know and love. There were people who offered a prayer in their churches. A friend's Muslim mother offered a special morning prayer. Buddhist friends offered to send positive energy. Other friends lit candles and offered warm thoughts and healing energy. My long-time friend and Reiki teacher Sister Eileen offered a complimentary reiki treatment and spent four hours talking to me. She assured me that in her heart, she felt there was going to be a miracle and that I was going to learn so much from this experience.

Appointment at the BC Cancer Agency

Immediate plan for chemotherapy and radiation

It was not long after my meeting with the neurosurgeon in Victoria that I received a call from the BC Cancer Agency scheduling me for appointments with the oncologist and radiologist for chemotherapy and radiation treatments. I was surprised by the rigidity and insensitivity of the woman who set the appointments. When I mentioned at first that I couldn't make one of the appointments due to a previous appointment set with a specialist in Vancouver, her response was "Why not?", and then she scolded me and gave me a lecture on how busy the oncologists are. She said that I was very fortunate to receive this appointment and needed to set my priorities straight and just take the appointments that I was given and cancel everything else.

Part of me wanted to scream as loud as I could, "Do you have any idea what it is like to be told YOU HAVE A MALIGNANT BRAIN TUMOR? In fact, do you even realize that you are working at the Cancer Agency and deal with people whose lives have been turned upside down with the news of having CANCER?" But I didn't. I, who once was able to sing opera in large theatres for hundreds of people without a microphone, could not even raise my voice. Instead, I softly responded that my appointment in Vancouver was with a neurosurgeon and I could not possibly cancel it. I asked her very nicely if she would be kind enough to give me another appointment. She hesitantly agreed and said she had to look at the schedule and call me back. To my surprise, she did call back a few minutes later and gave me another appointment for the following week.

The next week, Mina and I arrived at the BC Cancer Agency for the appointment. I went to the desk and said that I had an appointment with one of the oncologists. The young woman hardly acknowledged me, handed me a form and a pen, and said to fill it out and have a seat in the main lobby. I started to fill out the form. It was a new experience for me. Normally, I would go through the questions and just check the "no" boxes without even looking at the conditions; however, this time I had to be careful because there were some boxes where I had to say "yes."

As I waited, I observed all the people who were there and searched desperately for someone who looked relatively well. Surely, all these treatments with so much promise had to be working for someone. After all, didn't my own neurosurgeon tell me that chemotherapy was going to do wonders for my tumor? To my disappointment, I could not find anyone that looked well or even looked happy to be there. There were women with hats and wigs trying to look "normal." Some even put on makeup to cover up their pale complexions. Men tried to look heroic but they were also in the same predicament. The volunteers tried to cheer people up by offering free coffee and cookies. In fact, they were very much the life of the place.

Soon, a nurse called my name and Mina and I were ushered to a room to meet the oncologist. A few minutes later, a very nice doctor with a kind face walked into the room. After greetings, he proceeded to say that they had discussed my case in their meetings with the neurosurgeon and other oncologists, and the consensus was that surgery was not an option; therefore, the course of treatment was chemotherapy and then a round of radiation. He was very kind and talked with us for nearly an hour. He encouraged me to live my life as I did before (which I later understood to be the usual advice of all oncologists) and go back to teaching. I said I was prepared to take some time off to deal with this illness and treatments. Mina then added that she was also planning to take a few months off to help. Right away, I responded that I didn't want her to put her life on hold for me, at which point the oncologist looked at both of us and smiled and said it was very nice to see two sisters who are so supportive and concerned for the well-being of one another.

He handed me two sets of information sheets. The first one—he called this the "gold standard"—talked about a combination of three chemotherapy drugs called procarbazine, lomustine, and vincristine (PCV), which was used for malignant brain tumors. He called it the gold standard because it had been in use since the 1990s. The second set talked about temozolomide, which had been in use for the past few years. After receiving the information, we informed him that we were going to see a neurosurgeon in Vancouver for a second opinion. He applauded our decision and said that he would be more than happy to do whatever he could for me. Mina and I thanked him and left his office.

We came out and sat on a bench in the lobby and started to read the information we had received. Starting with the gold standard, aside from the first two pages, the package consisted of six pages of serious side effects, including not only the usual nausea, vomiting, and hair loss, but also a lower white blood cell count (which lowered the patient's immune system, making him/her more prone to infections), a lower platelet count (which reduced the ability for blood to clot, so even a simple cut could have severe consequences), numbness or tingling in fingers or toes, headaches, and dizziness. Other possible side effects included problems with the lungs, kidneys, liver, and skin as well as vision and hearing.

The side effects of the newer drug only covered one page, and only—yes, only—included effects on the blood cells leading to an increased risk of infection and bleeding.

I could feel my heart racing. Did I really want to go through with this? What quality of life would I have?

Also, more importantly, vision problems, hearing problems, and numbness in the fingers meant that teaching opera history, singing, playing the piano, and yoga were definitely out of the question. There was not even a remote possibility of going back to my earlier career of research, analysis, and project management. In fact, what would be left for me? Would that even be a life worth living?

Meeting the Neurosurgeon
in Vancouver

"No" to chemotherapy and radiation

An uneasy few weeks passed. I couldn't sleep much, as I contemplated the enormous challenge in front of me.

When I went to see my physician, I found out that even though the neurosurgeon in Victoria asked me not to show Dr. Kelly's note to the neurosurgeon in Vancouver in order to get an unbiased opinion, he had written a letter himself and sent a copy to the neurosurgeon in Vancouver as well as to my physician. The letter indicated that an aggressive removal of the tumor (as Dr. Kelly suggested) would bring a high risk of a deficit in the motor cortex area that may not improve over time. His letter further indicated the following:

"The risk of a left craniotomy would include but would not be limited to: infection/meningitis, hemorrhage, worsened seizures, the increased neurologic deficit, which would be permanent and would include hemiparesis or hemiplegia (paralysis of one side), language dysfunction or visual disturbance."

The letter continued, "If she wishes to proceed with the surgery in Victoria, I would be happy to accommodate her...."

I tried everything in my power to remain calm. My level of distrust in this neurosurgeon grew tenfold. To behave in such a manner, write such a letter, and then expect me to have my surgery with him? Were we even on the same planet? Truly, at this moment, the chance of me having this surgery with him was much less than being struck by lightning.

The day of my appointment with the neurosurgeon in Vancouver arrived. Mina and I had taken the bus the night before and stayed with Lila and her family. These nearly five-hour bus and ferry trips were becoming a regular occurrence for us. The next morning, Mina, Lila, and I got up early and soon were on our way to see the neurosurgeon. I was rehearsing what I was going to tell him in light of the letter that he had received.

He met the three of us and after introductions, accompanied us to his office. After we sat down, I talked about the fact that the neurosurgeon in Victoria had suggested to me that I not provide a copy of the second opinion I received, so that I would get an unbiased opinion at this appointment, but then had written a letter himself. This doctor smiled and calmly suggested that we start fresh, and then asked me to tell him everything from the beginning. So once again I told the familiar story, from my initial seizure episode at home to the present, and then talked about the two conflicting opinions of the neurosurgeons.

His first words were that in his opinion, chemotherapy and radiation were too aggressive to treat a grade II oligodendroglioma. He felt that in his experience, the side effects of radiation on the brain were irreversible, and the negative impacts of radiation on vision, hearing, and cognitive abilities could be permanent. I felt numb after hearing this, thinking how close I had come to being totally disabled and incapacitated.

However, he also said that he felt that the tumor was too close to my speech area, and with an aggressive surgery, there was a moderate risk of having speech problems, with full recovery being uncertain. Upon hearing that I teach and sing, he said this might be important for me to consider. He then asked if he could look at the incision of the biopsy. In an astonished tone, he said, "He opened the skull that much for a biopsy?!?" I froze for a moment and with no appropriate answer just looked at him and quietly responded that I had had 18 stitches.

In total disbelief, he shook his head and went back to his seat and said that in his opinion, if I elected to have the surgery I should have it in Vancouver, and for that matter, I should also have my MRIs done in Vancouver since the machines were much more accurate for the brain. In the end, he said that with the type of tumor I had—slow growing—the best thing would be to monitor it regularly with an MRI to measure the growth.

His last words to me were, "Just go ahead and enjoy your summer and don't worry about this and let me worry about it." Although at the time, I was touched emotionally by these words, I questioned afterwards if it was really possible for someone with a malignant brain tumor to "enjoy the summer" and not worry about their illness. Somehow, that did not seem possible to me.

We left his office more confused than ever. I asked Mina whether she remembered Dr. Kelly saying anything about speech problems when we had our conversation with him on the phone. She did not recall hearing anything related to speech. After what we had just heard, we were all unsure what would be the right thing to do. We sat in the building's lobby and looked at each other, stunned and uncertain.

At this time, all the plans had been made to go to Los Angeles. Everyone had reserved and paid for their airfare, we had found a house close to the hospital for all of us to stay, and with the date of the surgery booked, we were all set to leave for Los Angeles in a few days. We were headed back to Victoria the next day, and Lila was coming with us as well, since we were all booked on a flight to Los Angeles from Victoria.

On our way to Victoria, our minds went everywhere with ideas. Perhaps we should cancel the surgery and just go and see Dr. Kelly for a consultation. However, I remembered that Dr. Kelly had advised that I not put off the surgery for long. We went back and forth, and whether it was this uncertainty, or the fatigue from the trip, or just trying so hard to keep it together for so long, or a combination of everything, tears started to stream down my face. Mina and Lila came to my aid with words of encouragement. They said that I should listen to my intuition and in the end, it was my decision and I should not worry about anyone else but me. I was surrounded by all this amazing support and yet could not find the right answer.

Back in Victoria, I was about to cancel the surgery and make an appointment for a consultation, when all of a sudden Lila had a brilliant idea. She suggested that I call Dr. Kelly and ask him about the risk of speech problems.

Without hesitation, I called him and left a voicemail saying that I had an important question. It turned out that Dr. Kelly had a complicated case that day and spent nearly ten hours in surgery. It was 8:30 p.m. when the phone finally rang and it displayed the area code of Los Angeles. I answered it immediately and Dr. Kelly was on the line, apologizing for not getting back to me earlier. It was heartwarming to hear his calm and caring voice again. As coherently as I could, I tried to explain what the neurosurgeon in Vancouver had said about the surgery bringing with it the possibility of a moderate risk of speech problems, and asked him what he thought. He calmly asked if he could look at the MRI again and get back to me in ten minutes. I thanked him and said that I would wait for his phone call.

Before the ten minutes were over, the phone rang again. It was Dr. Kelly, and he said in his usual confident tone, "I completely disagree with this surgeon. There is at least one centimetre between your tumor and the speech area." I later learned that one centimetre in brain surgery is quite a distance. He was quick to point out that he was not forcing me to have surgery and it was completely up to me. To this, I responded that we had made all the arrangements and thanked him again for calling me at this time of the night, especially knowing that he had had a very difficult day. Again, his response was so typical of his amazing character, "Sometimes, you have days like that."

With no uncertainty left in my mind, we were soon on our way to Los Angeles.

The Coming of July 8th

The beginning of the journey of courage and hope

Our day of journey to Los Angeles had come. There was none of the excitement, laughter, or joy that usually accompanies the preparation for a trip. Instead, there was a heaviness accompanied by an uneasy anxiousness.

Lila tried her best to cheer me up and make me feel better. She insisted on doing my hair and was not bothered by my lack of enthusiasm as a result of the shaving of my hair from the biopsy. She put rollers in my hair to compensate for the obvious and to my surprise she was successful. She was no stranger to pain herself, as she had overcome a major illness a few years ago. However, she was always positive, with a wicked sense of humour that would stop even the most serious person in their tracks and make them burst into spontaneous laughter.

In the early hours of the morning, despite being weary, I decided again to remain positive. After all, it was my journey and I could either go through it with avoidance and anger or come to terms with it and accept it with peace and grace. Somehow, the latter seemed more hopeful.

We got to the airport and were soon on our first, short flight to Seattle. I tried to bury myself in Rilke's *Letters to a Young Poet*. In one part, he says how it is nearly impossible to explain certain experiences, as they seem to happen in a space without words. This echoed very much what I had been feeling for the past few months.

After a change of plane in Seattle, we soon arrived at the Los Angeles airport. We spotted my brothers-in-law, Farid and Mehdi, who were there to pick us up and take us to the house that was to be our home for the next two weeks. Although Mehdi was older than Farid and they lived so far apart, you would not have guessed this difference in age, judging by the way they talked and joked with each other. It was beautiful to experience this lightness, which took me away from my problems, albeit only momentarily.

After a short drive, we arrived at the house. Right away, I noticed the high ceilings and an upright piano in the corner of one of the rooms. As soon as I put my bags down, I went to the piano and ran my fingers across the keys. I contemplated what it would be like not to be able to play and quickly brought myself back to the present moment. For now, hope still remained.

By coincidence, the house belonged to a Persian couple; the fellow, an anaesthesiologist, happened to know Dr.

Kelly. As soon as he found out why we were there and heard that my surgeon was Dr. Kelly, he said that he had heard nothing but good things about Dr. Kelly. I took this as yet another sign that I had made the right decision.

Although the dining room table was beautifully set with fruits freshly picked by Sheila and Mehdi from their garden and salads so elegantly prepared by Roya, my thoughts were with the promise that I had made to Sholeh to call her as soon as I arrived. So I ate quickly and called her. After a brief conversation, we decided to meet for coffee the next day. My mind was anxiously racing to come to terms with meeting Sholeh. Who would have thought when we were not even teenagers, that we would be separated for so many years and then meet again under such unbelievable circumstances?

Catching Up with Sholeh
After Nearly 40 Years

I got up early that next morning, still rehearsing in my mind what it would be like to see Sholeh for the first time in 38 years. After breakfast, there was a knock at the door and soon Sholeh and I were in each other's arms, with tears flowing as predictably as west coast rain during the spring.

She took me to a café that she said was one of her favourite places. I don't remember anything about the place or the food. All I remember was being immersed in our conversations of the past and present, weaving our innocence with the hardship of being a teenager in a foreign land not knowing the language, and then facing challenges, including major illnesses. After two hours, we both felt that 38 years apart had not changed how we felt about each other and were amazed at how the universe had brought us together again under such surreal circumstances.

Sholeh was in awe of my peacefulness despite what I was going through. I told her that I owed it to my yoga students to practice what I had preached to them in terms of breathing deeply and engaging the parasympathetic nervous system, which was essentially responsible for the body's immune system. She asked if I would show her this way of breathing and I happily obliged. We laughed as we tried to breathe together while sitting in her car and wondered what people passing by would think of us. It soon came time to say goodbye. She held me tight and wished me well and said she would come to see me in the hospital after my surgery.

I got out of her car and walked to the door. I thought about whether my original idea of meeting her in a café somewhere in Europe would have been more memorable than this exchange that we just shared. The essence of seeing each other and sharing the difficulty of our illnesses after all these years brought a depth to our relationship that was so profound and almost indescribable.

Invitation from Jaleh and Feraidoon

That same evening, Sheila's friend Jaleh invited us to her apartment. I met her and her husband Feraidoon for the first time. The story of their friendship with Sheila and Mehdi went back over 25 years. The closeness between the four of them was evident from the first moment. The evening started with sharing life stories and adventures, some of which were truly unbelievable, but so telling of the bond between these four people.

Jaleh was originally trained as a nurse. While she worked as a nurse, she went back to university to do her Ph.D. and now was in charge of the surgical rooms in the hospital. She explained what was going to happen with the surgery and we all listened intently. She did everything possible to set our minds at ease and her confident tone and demeanour conveyed exactly what we all so eagerly wanted to hear.

Jaleh's husband Feraidoon was a musician and played several instruments beautifully. He had worked with some very well respected classical Iranian singers and had a personality and sense of humour that would light up any room and atmosphere. Soon, the living room was turned into a music studio as both Feraidoon and Mehdi asked me to sing *Che farò senza Euridice?* This is an aria from the opera *Orfeo ed Euridice*, where Orfeo, having lost his wife, laments on living life without his beloved. This happened to be the absolute favourite piece for both Feraidoon and Mehdi. I started to sing with complete abandon, as if it was my last opportunity to sing. After I finished, I saw a precious glimpse of an emotional exchange between Feraidoon and Mehdi, who looked at each other with tears in their eyes. I thought how fortunate I was to experience this moment, even if this was to be perhaps my last time singing.

The evening continued with more music as Feraidoon played his tar and everyone lent their voices to songs and expressions of joy. Although no one wanted this evening to end, it was getting late and we all decided it was time to leave. Before leaving, I gave Jaleh and Faraidoon my cd of Spanish songs that I had recorded a few years earlier.

Pre-Operation Tests and
Meeting Dr. Kelly

The next day, I had an appointment for an MRI and other tests prior to the surgery and also had my first consultation with Dr. Kelly. My family decided to accompany me, which was very touching knowing that this was going to be a very long and uninteresting day.

Soon I was called in for the MRI. I decided to try something new this time so the sound would not bother me as much. Generally, MRIs for the brain take longer, because halfway through, they inject a dye intravenously to show the contrast and see a clearer diagnostic image. I thought about what I could possibly do to make the sound not affect me as much. As soon as I heard the repetitive sounds, I tried to think of what piece of music would go with them and suddenly, I remembered Beethoven's Ode to Joy from his 9th Symphony. I sang the choral piece to myself over and over again and before I knew it, I heard the voice of the technician telling me that there were only a few minutes left. Afterward, I thought how ironic it was that Beethoven was totally deaf when he composed this masterpiece. Indeed, knowing the amazing man he was, how would he have felt if he knew that his music would be helping a woman in such a dire situation nearly 200 years later?

After the MRI, we went for my appointment with Dr. Kelly. Mina, Sheila, and Jaleh were with me as Dr. Kelly walked in the room. His voice and demeanour were as calm as the Pacific Ocean on a summer day. He explained what was going to take place and asked if he had answered all my questions and concerns with regards to possible speech problems. I was very touched that he had remembered our previous phone conversation. I responded favourably and said with a smile "I am here!" At this point, he asked how I was feeling and if I had any other questions. Before I could answer, Jaleh replied that I was calm enough to sing a couple of pieces for them the night before. I thought this was the perfect segue way for me to give him my cd of Spanish songs. I took the cd out of my bag and gave it to him, saying that I had discovered from Jaleh that he spoke Spanish and that his wife was Spanish, so I thought they would enjoy listening to a cd of Spanish songs that I had recorded a few years ago. He looked at the cd with great interest and said, "Wow, this is you!" pointing to my name on the cd cover. I replied that it was me, and went on to explain that I had recorded it a few years ago after finishing a music program in Granada, Spain.

He smiled and said, "Gracias."

I also smiled and replied, "De nada."

He put the cd carefully in the pocket of his lab coat and asked us if we had any further questions. The room was quiet so he pleasantly said goodbye and said that he would see us on the day of the surgery.

The day continued with more blood tests, an EKG, and chest x-ray. The woman who did my EKG was a gentle and sweet middle-aged African American with a distinct southern accent. She asked me, "So, honey, who is your surgeon?" When I replied that it was Dr. Kelly, she said right away, "Dr. Kelly is the best. You are in the greatest hands honey and don't have anything to worry about." I thanked her and said that I felt the same.

The day ended with all of us having dinner at a famous Persian restaurant. As we all enjoyed the fine cuisine, I thought how fortunate I was to be surrounded by so much love and support, even though, at times, without even being conscious of it, my mind would go to the dark side of fear and worry and I had to distract myself and bring it back to focus on the present.

The next day was spent just relaxing and getting ready for the day of the surgery. We decided to go for short walks and a coffee and to go to bed early as we were told to arrive at the hospital no later than 6:30 a.m. the following day.

The Day of the Surgery

The next morning, we were all up, dressed, and out the door by 5:30 a.m. The absurdity of being on the street at such a time was shown by the empty streets in the heart of Los Angeles, a city known for its heavy traffic not only at rush hour but also at most times of the day.

There was absolute silence in the car, which was quite unusual for us. Clearly, everyone was preoccupied with thoughts of what was to come. I was calm and tried to feel my breath low in my belly as if I was about to go on stage and sing a full program of songs and arias. Well, perhaps in a way I was.

When we arrived at the hospital, I registered at the desk and was told to go and wait in a room full of patients that were about to go for surgery. Soon, a nurse called my name and told my sisters that they could join me momentarily. I was asked to put on a gown and just sit on the bed. Shortly after, Jaleh came in and she looked so striking in her red suit, which contrasted so beautifully against her shoulder-length gray hair. I complimented her on her look and she gave me a surprised look. I don't think she expected to see me so relaxed and able to

85

notice and comment on such things. She soon introduced me to the anaesthesiologist, a very kind woman who told me what was going to happen and asked if I wanted to hear what could possibly go wrong. I replied that I didn't want to hear that—what good would come out of hearing the negative, and why not just go with a positive outlook and hope for the best?

At this point, Jaleh said that she was going to change into her scrubs and then come and be with me during the surgery. I was very touched by this overwhelming gesture of kindness. And then my family came into the room and embraced me one by one and I could feel how each and every one of them tried so hard to hide their anxious feelings. After all, it was one thing going through a major brain surgery and totally another to watch someone you love go through it.

I could now feel that I was getting drowsy as a result of the anaesthetic. I was awake enough to see Jaleh come back into the room and hold my hand as I was wheeled into the operating room.

Next thing I remembered was waking up in the recovery room. As I slowly opened my eyes, I could hear a conversation between two nurses. The young woman who was sitting and watching me was asked if she wanted to take a break, knowing that her father had just been brought into the emergency room with a possible heart attack. She calmly responded that she was okay and that she wanted to sit with me. I opened my eyes and the first thing I did was to move my right hand and right leg.

The nurse asked me how I was and I replied with an answer that she understood perfectly—this meant that there were no problems with my speech. Suddenly, even the smallest movements and actions brought euphoria beyond imagination. Before long, tears of joy were streaming down my face. Seeing my tears, the nurse asked me if I was in pain, and I replied that I was just overjoyed with the results of the surgery. She smiled and said that I could have a visit from one family member at a time. Who did I want to see first? I asked to see Mina. Poor Mina was so worried when she saw my tears but I soon explained that I was joyous that everything was working. Soon after, each and every member of my family came and embraced me, all of them crying tears of joy. This was an incredible moment for all of us, for it brought into perspective what was truly the most important element in life: the ability to feel, express, and share all emotions, perhaps the most beautiful qualities of human beings.

After some time, the young nurse was told that I was ready to be taken from the recovery room to the critical care unit. I asked if she was coming with me and she said yes. When we were in the room alone, I held her hand and said that I would send healing thoughts to her father. She looked at me in total amazement. I continued to hold her hand, looked into her eyes and said, "Stay strong," and at that moment her eyes filled with tears, she kissed my hand and said, "You too." Soon after, upon seeing my family enter the room, she left.

My small, private room was soon filled with members of my family, and I was so happy to see them again. Soon after, Sholeh came and was crying, not able to believe how well I looked considering what I had been through. Later, Dr. Kelly came into the room and asked how I was feeling. I said fine, at which moment he turned to Sholeh to shake hands and introduce himself. Sholeh looked at him with a smile and said "You don't recognize me?" to which he responded, "Oh yes, of course, how do the two of you know each other?" We explained that we had reconnected after nearly 40 years and we had both had our surgeries with him. A look of amazement was apparent on his face. I heard later that he talked about us at his meeting with the other surgeons.

After everyone left, I noticed a big apparatus attached to my left hand that made it hard for me to lift it. When I asked a nurse about it, she explained that apparently, my blood pressure was low during the surgery so they had to elevate it with some medication, and now they needed to monitor me constantly to ensure that my blood pressure returned to normal.

I looked at the clock in front of me and it showed 6:15 p.m. Exactly 12 hours had passed since the surgery that the other two surgeons thought would be too risky and nearly impossible to do, and as far as I could tell, I was still able to think, understand, speak, and move my right hand and leg. For me, this was a substantial victory given my initial prognosis.

I also couldn't help but compare how I felt after this surgery compared to my biopsy. There was a dim light on in the room and the nurses' station was just across from me, and yet I was not bothered at all by the sounds of pagers and phones going off, not to mention the sound of all the machines that were attached to me. My mind went back to how I felt in the first room after my biopsy, when the sound of the book coming out of the plastic bag was like thunder and lightning. The surgery I had just experienced was three times longer than the biopsy and obviously a lot more complicated. Was the difference in how I felt explained by the difference in the skill and experience of the neurosurgeons? At this point, I lifted my right hand, moved my fingers, opened and closed each and every one, and in absolute awe, put my hand on my heart, sent a message of gratitude to Dr. Kelly, and closed my eyes.

A half-hour later, the nurse came to check on me and asked if I needed anything. She watched me with amazement as I used my right hand to successfully pour water from the jug into a plastic cup located on my right side. I smiled with a sense of pride and brought the plastic cup and straw close to my lips. The sensation of the cool water on my tongue and throat was indescribable. I thought for a moment how much we take for granted as human beings.

I didn't get much sleep throughout the night. There was a head trauma case that came in during the night and demanded the close attention of all the doctors and nurses. It was interesting that all this commotion did not bother me a bit. I only had to ask for pain medication once, and I was happy that every time I opened my eyes, I didn't have the delusions as I did after the biopsy. This proved to me that Dr. Cameron was correct about the morphine allergy. Once again, I couldn't help but think how much of a comfort it was for me to remember Montserrat Caballé's *Signore, ascolta* during those dark times. And how even imagining her singing the final note would make my heart skip a beat.

The Morning After the Surgery

The next morning, I heard the sound of a wheelchair coming to my room. An attendant said that he was taking me for a post-operative MRI. I was surprised to see the wheelchair; he had obviously been told that I was able to stand and sit in a wheelchair. He brought the wheelchair very close to the bed. To my surprise, I was able to put one foot on the floor and then the other, and, with his help, stand up, turn, and sit in the wheelchair. No gift was greater for me at that moment.

As I was wheeled through the bare, white hallway, I felt that this was the most beautiful place on earth. There was nothing greater for me than being given the gift of walking, moving, seeing, hearing, thinking, understanding, and being aware of everything that was taking place around me. I could feel the tears welling up in my eyes as I was positioned on the MRI bed with a device holding my head in place. In the privacy of the MRI tunnel, I could feel the sensation of gentle teardrops leaving the corners of my eyes, moistening the side of my face like morning dew on a rose petal on the first day of spring, reflecting a rebirth and a new beginning. I was immersed in these thoughts and feelings when suddenly I heard that the MRI session was finished. I was brought out of the MRI tunnel and again I was able to stand and sit back in the wheelchair to return to my room.

When I arrived at my room I saw Jaleh, who had come to check on me. She said that everything went as expected with the surgery, and she was so happy to see me doing so well. I knew that she had stopped by to see me before she started her very busy day and I was so touched by her kindness. I held her hand and thanked her and she smiled and said she would stop by to see me before the end of the day. At this time, a new nurse came in and informed me that I was being transferred to the post-critical care unit, which meant that my situation was no longer critical. I was very pleased to hear this news.

My Stay at the Post-Critical Care Unit

I looked at the clock and it was shortly before 8:00 a.m. With the night I had had, I was ready for a good rest. There was still plenty of time before friends and family came to visit so I rested my head and closed my eyes.

Suddenly, I felt the presence of a young woman who came in and introduced herself as my occupational therapist. With a walker in hand, she informed me that she was about to take me for a walk. I questioned how this could be possible—standing up and sitting in a wheelchair was one thing but now she wanted me to go for a walk? I asked her, "You mean going for a walk now?" She replied, "Absolutely! But first, we are going to stand." Seeing her enthusiasm and determination, I didn't think she would take a "maybe later" for an answer, so as tired as I was, I decided to try and see what happened. I followed her instructions and sat at the edge of the bed and put my feet on the floor. With her help, I stood and she looked at me in absolute disbelief. She said, "Wow, this is amazing. I think you can actually do this without a walker!" At this moment, she slowly let go of my hands one by one and I stood on my own.

My heart began to beat faster than usual and I needed to remind myself to breathe deeper and calm down. She instructed me to take one step and then another and before I knew it, we were past the door and into the circular hallway. I could feel the heaviness of my head but was overjoyed at being able to walk, albeit very slowly.

All of sudden, I heard a male voice calling my name very loud from the other side of the hallway, pronouncing it beautifully. At first, I thought it was perhaps either Mehdi or Farid, yet I knew it was too early for them to be at the hospital. Very slowly, I turned my head towards the right and to my absolute surprise saw Dr. Kelly! I smiled and said hello and his face was beaming with joy to see me walking. He was far away and I slowly walked towards him. He gestured and said that I should continue my walk with the occupational therapist and that he would come and see me shortly. I slowly turned around and continued to walk but somehow knew that I would never forget this moment, which involved an exchange of just a few words but communicated volumes of emotion and feelings.

Before I knew it, we had finished our walk and had arrived back at my room. The occupational therapist congratulated me and said that she would be back the next day to show me what I needed to know before being discharged.

I was resting in bed and contemplating what had just taken place when Dr. Kelly walked in and offered his hand, which I held with both of mine in a gesture of respect and gratitude. He calmly said that based on my pre-operative MRI, he was able to remove around 90 percent of the tumor and essentially everything was in my favour. He said that they had sent the tumor to the pathology lab and were waiting for the results. I smiled and expressed my gratitude to him as best as I could, for words truly failed me at this moment. What can you say to someone who not only saved your life but also your identity and who you are as a human being? To my small expression of gratitude, he offered his gentle smile and left the room, saying that he looked forward to seeing me the next day.

I looked around the room and saw an alcove with a window. I imagined myself sitting there and writing in my journal, recording these profound and beautiful moments that I knew one day I would look back on as great memories. While I couldn't quite conceive of holding a pen in my hand at this moment, even the real possibility of it warmed my heart. As I was reflecting on what had taken place in the past 24 hours and how it was going to change my life in such a remarkable way, my family walked in. I was showered with kisses and hugs and an abundance of home-cooked meals and fresh fruits. Feraidoon, Jaleh's husband, also came for a visit. He held my right hand with such tenderness and with tears in his eyes said how happy he was to see me doing so well. It was so beautiful and touching beyond belief. I wanted to embrace everyone and just hold onto all this beauty around me, but as enthusiastic as I tried to be, my physical body was feeling the fatigue and sheer exhaustion of the surgery, so I found it very hard to keep my eyes open. Everyone respected my needs and left the room quickly.

A few hours later, I saw Jaleh again as she stopped by to see me before she left the hospital to go home. She said everyone on the medical team was so happy to see me doing so well. I thanked her for being there with me from the beginning. She very humbly replied that she didn't do anything special. As she said goodbye, I could see the clear signs of a full day of an enormously responsible position on her face. I thought about how many cases like mine she had handled in her long career and how enormously rewarding it must have been for her to see patients go through difficult surgeries and come out feeling so well. The lights dimmed, indicating the coming of the time of rest for patients. With little hesitation, my heavy eyelids brought an end to this incredible day.

My Second Day at the Post-Critical Care Unit

The day started early, with the nurse coming to measure my blood pressure and then give me a wash and change of gown. As promised, the occupational therapist came in to watch me as I did my morning routine of washing my face and brushing my teeth. I was so grateful and proud to be able to do these things that I had taken for granted all my life. As I revelled in the fact that I was able to do all of this, I thought about how interesting we are as human beings. More often than not, we do not even contemplate how much we are able to do and often complain when some little thing goes wrong. I thought about how much this illness had already altered the way I thought about life and what was truly important.

As soon as I was back in bed, a woman from the kitchen came to ask for my food order. She told me about the main dishes and expected me to choose from the menu that she was listing. The varied menu included a chicken dish, and fish or beef with potatoes and vegetables. For some reason, nothing appealed to me except fresh fruit, so I asked if I could have a fruit plate. She kindly informed me that the fruit was usually served as dessert.

I asked if I could possibly have a dinner plate filled with all kinds of different fruits. She looked at me as I described this plate of fruit and salivated over sounding out the names of grapes, blueberries, cantaloupe, and watermelon. She stopped me and said that she would do her best to get me what I had asked for. I started to laugh to myself and imagined the possible conversations among the kitchen staff about the request from the strange woman on the second floor who had just had brain surgery!

Soon after, a few members of my family arrived for a visit. Dr. Kelly came to visit me at the same time. He was happy to see everyone and took time to say hello to them all. He said he was very pleased with my progress. He examined the incision, mentioning that he had followed the same incision as the biopsy, and said he was pleased that it was healing well. I took the opportunity to ask—mainly to satisfy my own curiosity—whether he thought that this was a big incision for a biopsy. He just looked at the ceiling and shook his head. Although he didn't say anything, his reaction spoke volumes. I thanked him again and Mina looked at him and said, "You must have golden hands." He humbly replied, "I just do this all the time"—yet another affirmation of the character of this remarkable doctor and human being. He said that I should be discharged the following day and that he looked forward to seeing me in a week in his office.

Before long, the physical therapist, a very humorous African-American man, came into the room and informed us that in the hospital he was known as "the King of Balance"! Essentially he was famous for challenging people with their balance. For the moment, I decided to keep the fact that I was a yoga teacher to myself. He began by taking me for a walk and asking me to walk in a straight line forward and back with my eyes closed. And then he said, "Now comes the challenging part. I am now going to ask you to stand on one leg."

I replied, "Would you like me to do the tree pose for you?"

Looking somewhat perplexed, he replied, "What is that?"

Without saying a word, in the middle of the hallway, I went into the tree pose, first on the right leg and then on the left. And then I revealed to him that I had been a yoga practitioner and a teacher for a few years. He was quite impressed. As he was about to take me back to my room, my sister Sheila asked if he thought I could easily go up and down the stairs, as we were staying in a house that had a few stairs. He smiled and replied, "Well, ladies, we could certainly try the stairs to ease your mind. I know she would be ok (pointing to me); I am not sure about me and the rest of you!" So we went to the stairway at the back of the hallway, and now I was faced with a set of ten to fifteen steps that I had to navigate. At the same time, he asked my sisters to come up the stairs with me. With so much at stake, I took a deep breath and calmly started to climb the stairs. To my surprise, I was not even out of breath and I could see everyone else, including the physical therapist, breathing heavily. Proudly, as if this was nothing, I came down the stairs. As he brought me back to my room, the physical therapist congratulated me and said I was more than ready to be discharged the next day. Soon after, one of the nurses came in and said, "I heard you showed the physical therapist how to walk!" We all laughed.

Shortly after the physical therapy session, all my sisters left and I was back in bed resting. I looked over at my side table and found my journal and favourite fountain pen. I thought I would make my way slowly to the alcove in my room, put a pillow behind my back, and start to write. I was hesitant to write at first, but was determined to try and see what happened. I took off the top of the pen, opened my journal and began to write. First the date, then the first sentence, then the second, and soon I could see my handwriting was as fine as ever. The pen glided on the paper with hardly any effort, writing words and sentences that were full of the true sentiments of the moment. Suddenly the words became blurry as my eyes filled with tears. I stopped and looked at my hand— my right hand—still capable of doing what my brain was telling it to do. What gift could be greater for me at this very moment?

And then this beautiful moment was interrupted by yet another beautiful moment, as Mehdi and Roya came to visit me in the evening. We had an amazing conversation about life, its tragedies, and triumphs. They stayed and watched me enjoy the beautiful plate of fruit that was brought for me. It was exactly as I imagined it, filled with the best fresh fruits of the season.

Release from the Hospital and
Recuperation at Home in Los Angeles

After being released from the hospital, I spent another week in our rented house with my family before a post-operative appointment with Dr. Kelly and Dr. Kesari, the neuro-oncologist. My first few days were spent at the house resting and recuperating. Every once in a while, I had to remind myself of how this all could have turned out. I would then close my eyes and slowly open them, looking at my surroundings, freely moving my hands, arms, and legs, thinking, understanding, and saying a few words to myself, just to make sure that this was not just a beautiful dream—and no, it was not a dream.

It was not even a week after my surgery and I was able to do everything without anyone's help. There were many moments of joyful exchanges, but a particular one that stayed with me was with Mehdi one morning in the kitchen. We were both standing waiting for the kettle to boil for tea when he looked at me and expressed his happiness at how good I looked. He said that if he didn't know it, he would not believe that I had even had such a major surgery. I thanked him graciously and said jokingly that all he had to do to be sure was to look at the stitches on my head. To this, he replied that I could easily set a new fashion trend with all the body piercings that were happening these days. I could not help but smile at him, for whether he intended it or not, he created a beautiful memory for me forever.

After a few days of resting at home, Sholeh called and asked if I would be up to going for dinner to celebrate. I gladly accepted. She said she would come and pick me up and then suggested that we go to one of her favourite restaurants in downtown Los Angeles.

After finding a long line up and a possible hour wait at that and another restaurant, we were ready to give up, but then we came across a relatively new vegan restaurant named Gratitude. They had a few empty tables so we were seated right away. I was quite intrigued by the restaurant's name. As we sat down, the server greeted us. Normally, the server would mention the specials of the day; to our surprise, she said that their theme of the day was for patrons to acknowledge someone. Sholeh and I looked at each other and said at the same time, "We don't even have to think about this one...Dr. Kelly!" The server gave us a confused look, so we explained how we found each other after nearly 40 years and both of us had had brain surgery with the same surgeon. The server said that she got shivers up and down her spine listening to our incredible story.

During the evening, Sholeh and I reminisced about what had taken place and how this amazing event had brought us together. We talked about how important it is to know that both of us had been given a second chance at participating fully in life and what we needed to do now was to truly live each moment.

Paul Kalanithi's
When Breath Becomes Air

B ack in Victoria, while I was making plans to come to Los Angeles, I met a friend; a very well-respected yoga teacher who I felt would provide space for me to share my recent diagnosis with her. After listening to my story and my decision to go to Los Angeles to have the surgery, she asked me if I had read the book *When Breath Becomes Air*. Seeing my negative response, she mentioned that the book was about a neurosurgeon who had, unfortunately, been diagnosed with stage IV lung cancer. Although the book was about his life from his adolescence and his love of literature, a good portion of it was about his experiences as a neurosurgeon.

My friend warned me that I should be judicious in deciding when to begin reading this book. Intrigue and curiosity took hold and I decided to order it and have it shipped to my sister Roya in Dallas. I asked her to bring it with her to Los Angeles. She gave me the book before the surgery, but I promised myself that I would not open it until after the surgery.

On my fourth day out of the hospital, I was up at 4:30

a.m. as I couldn't sleep. I didn't want to disturb anyone, so I got up quietly, picked up the book, and went into our bedroom's walk-in closet—which by many standards would equate to a small room! I was able to put a chair in there and sit comfortably with the help of a few pillows. I then turned on the light and began to read.

I became engrossed in the book, not only by the author's captivating writing, but also—more importantly—by his special qualities. From reading the book, it seemed he had a passion for writing first before he heard his calling to become a neurosurgeon. As I read about his ideas and his curiosity about the human brain, I was mesmerized by this truly extraordinary person.

After the first few pages where he described his own diagnosis of advanced lung cancer at such a young age, he talked about his childhood. He was fortunate enough to be introduced to classic literature at a young age and continued that curiosity and love of learning to higher education. His fascination with ideas and how the brain is able to process and adjudicate them led him to study medicine and become a neurosurgeon. He wrote that when he began to practice medicine, he noted the immense challenge for a patient (or family member) who is facing brain surgery, because of the very real possibility of debilitating physical and mental disabilities that could result in the loss of the patient's identity and humanity.[2]

---

[2] Paul Kalanithi, *When Breath Becomes Air* (New York: Random House, 2016).

In fact, when dealing with the brain, we are talking not only about the risk of losing the function of a limb or one's vision or hearing, but also about the risk of losing one's cognitive ability, memory, and ability to learn, understand, process and differentiate ideas, and communicate, all of which are core to who we are as human beings. Once these are taken away from a person, they become a prisoner of a society that they can't fully participate in—all due to the crime of being diagnosed with a brain tumor.

Later in the book, Kalanithi wrote about the primary motor cortex and how even minor damage during surgery could cause paralysis in the affected side of the body. He described the parts in the left side of the brain known as Broca and Wernicke, which are responsible for producing and understanding language respectively.[3] Any damage to Broca's area would result in a person losing the ability to speak, although they would still be able to understand others. On the other hand, any damage to Wernicke's area would result in the loss of the ability to understand language; although the person would still be able to speak, their speech would consist of sentences and phrases with no sense or context. Damage to both areas would result in the person becoming mute.[4]

At this point, I couldn't stop the tears from falling on the page, for he was telling my story. I imagined for a

---

[3] Named after the French neurosurgeon Paul Broca, and the German neurologist Carl Wernicke, who discovered the function of these two areas in the 1860s and 1870s respectively.

[4] Paul Kalanithi, *When Breath Becomes Air* (New York: Random House, 2016).

moment what my life would have been like if I didn't have the ability to speak, or if I spoke and nothing made sense, or worse yet, if I were completely mute. All of these cases would have resulted in an unbearable situation. Aside from the fact that I would not have been able to share my love of music and yoga with my students and all those who called me a passionate singer and a gifted teacher, I would be completely isolated from my family, friends, and society. With all my learning and experience, I could only offer silence to a society that communicates through language. I contemplated for a moment what kind of a life that would have been for me—a life without language would not be worth living.

I looked up at the window in front of me. The coming of dawn showed that more than four hours had passed. For the entire time, I had been reading this incredible book by this special person, who, in his short life, left such a legacy and touched so many lives—perhaps more than he himself ever imagined.

* * * * *

It was the day before the post-operative appointments. After lunch and a short stroll on the street, we returned home and had tea in the living room. I was enjoying the aroma of the earl gray tea that I was holding and was about to have my first sip when Mehdi came in and sat beside me. He very quietly asked if I would sing his favourite aria for him. Surprised, I asked, "You mean right now?" He replied, "Why not?"

I was quite hesitant, since this was not a simple song that I could just toss off, but a major operatic aria in Italian! For a moment, I weighed the risk of failure: What if the notes would not come as they should or even the words? What would that do not only to me but also to my biggest fans and supporters sitting and anxiously waiting in the living room? I thought for a moment and then decided to throw caution to the wind. I slowly put my cup of tea on the table and sat at the edge of the chair and said to myself just start on a note—any note since there was no accompaniment—and fly. And fly I did! I began to sing, and soon the right words and notes with the correct intonations were floating in the air, with my voice filling the high-ceilinged living room that felt like an enormous cathedral. There was no effort; everything was happening naturally and beautifully, and I was free to express the emotions of the piece. After I finished, the applause and the joy on everyone's face was truly unforgettable. I closed my eyes and knew that what I had experienced was a moment I would never forget.

Post-Operative Appointments

The next morning, we had an appointment with Dr. Kesari, the neuro-oncologist. He informed us that the lab results showed that the entire tumor was a grade II oligodendroglioma, and since over 90 percent of it was successfully removed, he thought the most reasonable option would be to monitor it for now by doing regular MRIs every three months. I thought for a moment to my day in Victoria where I was scheduled for chemotherapy and radiation, and how close I had come to being quite possibly mentally and physically disabled. The image of my brain on the computer screen showed a hole where the brain tumor was and just a slight residue of the tumor remained.

Later, we saw Dr. Kelly, who agreed with Dr. Kesari's approach and said he was looking forward to seeing my MRI in three months. I was not sure exactly what to say. Words somehow could not express how I felt at that moment. I remember I shook Dr. Kelly's hand and said thank you. Coming down the stairs from his office, I asked myself what was really meant by these two small words that came out of my mouth. Did they really express what was truly in my heart?

We all left Los Angeles the next day to three different destinations: San Diego, Dallas, and Victoria. For me and perhaps for all of us, it was an end, but also a new beginning.

Back in Victoria

Being at home brought me to a new reality. I had to try and grasp what had taken place in the last two weeks. I walked around my apartment doing everything I had done before my illness, and I was in awe of how well I felt. One day, I felt so compelled to write a letter of gratitude to Dr. Kelly. I started to write and the words just filled the page without conscious thought, as if they were coming from the deepest place in my heart.

Dear Dr. Kelly:

It has been just a week that I am back home in Victoria, BC and I feel compelled to write you. Nearly one week after the surgery, we were all sitting in our home away from home (rented house in Santa Monica (Los Angeles) when Mehdi (Sheila's husband) asked me to sing his favourite aria from the opera Orfeo ed Euridice. It was the first time that I would be singing (especially a piece that I have not often performed or is in my regular repertoire) so I hesitantly agreed. I started to sing and soon the right words and notes with correct intonations were floating in the air with my voice filling the room. There was no effort, I was just being part of the experience and was free in my ability to express the emotions of the piece. This was truly astonishing, especially as I shared

111

with you before, two surgeons in Canada told me that there would be a moderate risk that I wouldn't be able to speak properly for a year, let alone sing so you can't imagine how this felt for me on that very special day, which I will remember for the rest of my life.

As you know, my friend Sholeh (who also had her surgery with you) and I found each other after nearly 40 years. A few days after the surgery, we decided to go for dinner to celebrate. After we tried a few places and were told the wait time for a table would be nearly an hour, we came to a new vegan restaurant, which was called Gratitude. Our server mentioned to us that the theme of the day is whom we would like to acknowledge that day. Sholeh and I both looked at each other and said at the same time..."we don't even have to think about this one...Dr. Kelly!" When we mentioned our story to the server, she said she got shivers down her spine.

I just finished reading Paul Kalanithi's book, When Breath Becomes Air, a beautifully written book that is not only a story of hope and courage but gives one a respect and appreciation for the work that the brain surgeons do on a regular basis. As Paul Kalanithi says: Brain surgeons don't just save a life, they save a person's identity. Indeed, you strive to preserve people's passions, interests, what makes us unique without which we would only exist and not really be alive.

So I am eternally grateful to you for preserving my ability to learn, understand and explore new ideas, which is the quality that I love most about myself. In a few weeks, I will start to teach opera history but also therapeutic yoga. I always talked about the connection between deep breaths and engaging the parasympathetic nervous system to my students but never experienced the true impact of it until now. So many people have asked how I was able to go through such a major surgery being so much at peace? The answer is I put my trust in you and just concentrated on deep breathing and being positive.

I will explore the relationship between the brain and yoga further as I continue studying yoga therapy.

Wishing you a most beautiful day and…thank you.

In gratitude, Zhila

Not even an hour had passed before I received a response from Dr. Kelly:

Zhila, this is so sweet and nice of you. We are so happy you are doing well. Very happy to hear you are doing well back home in Victoria. And yes I know Café Gratitude – great place! And Marta and I love your CD of songs!

Would you mind if I share this note with the team?

Please stay in touch!

I read his response over and over again, as I found that it revealed so many different layers. This was a touching, compassionate, and heartfelt response from a brilliant neurosurgeon who managed to find time in his busy schedule to respond to a note from a patient, but it was also evident that he saw me as a human being and not just a case. Dr. Kelly truly heard my voice, and not just on the cd. He heard my inner voice, which so desperately needed to be heard—a voice that spoke of my identity, my values, the true essence of who I was and what I held to be so vital as a human being. And as he said in his short video on his website, he did treat me like I was a member of his family. Those of us who have been in this situation know so well how incredibly important it is to be heard, as we often feel that our voice, and perhaps our humanity, has been taken away by these serious illnesses.

Through my apartment window, I could see that autumn was fast approaching and with it the start of another year of teaching. As I reviewed my notes, I remembered when it all began: *The day before...Listening to Montserrat Caballé singing Signore, ascolta while driving to teach a course on Voices in Opera at the university...*

Without any hesitation, I decided to listen to Caballé's *Signore, ascolta*. The voice was still beautiful and her technical ability was still astonishing; however, this time, I heard something else that was so ethereal and visionary. I heard a deeper message of humanity; a revealing fact that we are all touched by gentleness, kindness, and the need for our voices to be heard, particularly when we are at our most vulnerable. And having gone through this experience with such a positive outcome, perhaps I was the one with the voice who needed to carry the torch for others...Signore, ascolta!

Nearly Two Years Later

It is now June 2019, nearly two years after my surgery. My recent MRI has shown that the remainder of the tumor is stable. I am now back doing everything I used to do before my diagnosis, although my approach to everything has changed. I have done research into nutrition, exercise, yoga, and meditation. More importantly, I have changed my approach to stress. Life still presents its challenges, but it is the thought process of dealing with these challenges that needed to change. I have also learned to be present in every experience, whether it is eating an apple or teaching a class full of people. No one really knows when his or her last day is on this planet, so for now, I will try to be in the moment as much as I can, help others, and fill my life with meaningful and precious moments.

The Reality of Brain Tumors

The incidence rate of malignant brain tumors (low- and high-grade gliomas including glioblastoma multiforme [grade IV], anaplastic astrocytoma [grade III], oligodendroglioma, and other sub types) is approximately one percent of all cancers in Canada and the United States. In fact, each year, only 6 to 8 people per 100,000 are diagnosed with a malignant brain tumor in both countries, compared to nearly 56 per 100,000 for lung cancer and nearly 125 per 100,000 for breast cancer. So naturally and understandably, there are many centres in Canada and the United States with outstanding care for these more common types of cancers, and not as many that can provide the right type of surgeries and care for malignant brain tumors.

If you or a family member is diagnosed with a brain tumor, it is of utmost importance to research and find a surgeon and supporting medical team with expertise in this area. Since my own diagnosis, I have heard of so many unfortunate disabilities and sometimes deaths that have occurred in both Canada and the United States. You owe it to yourself and your loved ones to take the time and do thorough research, and get a second or even a third opinion if necessary. Here are some of the things you can do:

- Take the first 48 hours after your diagnosis to digest the news. Give yourself permission to be totally emotional.

- After the initial 48 hours, it is important to research and learn as much as you can about your particular tumor. Please ensure that your sources are reliable. The Internet can often provide great information, but can also provide misinformation. There are many places to find reliable information. One of these is the Pacific Neuroscience Institute. The Institute's website contains a section on patient resources that is quite informative. Please visit: **https://www.pacificneuroscienceinstitute.org**

- Find a centre that has expertise in the area of neurosurgery and prepare a set of questions and concerns to ask the neurosurgeon. A compassionate neurosurgeon will take the time to answer all your questions. In particular, make sure you ask the neurosurgeon how many similar surgeries he/she performs per year. The expertise usually comes with experience.

- Take care of yourself. Pay attention to your diet, exercise, sleep, and stress level. The more you take care of yourself physically and emotionally, the more you are prepared for the challenging journey that faces you.

Expressions of Gratitude

I am grateful to a number of individuals who supported me throughout this challenging experience and also encouraged me to write about it.

First and foremost, I would like to thank Dr. Kelly. You are not only a brilliant neurosurgeon but also a remarkable human being and I am forever grateful to you for what you did for me. I am also grateful for the care of the team of doctors, nurses, staff, as well as the physiotherapist and occupational therapist while I was in the hospital for my surgery. I was so fortunate to be a patient at your facility and will recommend it to anyone in my situation.

My special thanks to Jaleh, the Director of Surgical Procedures, who not only introduced me to Dr. Kelly, but also tenderly accompanied me in the surgery room and came to see me every day while I was in the hospital. Your compassion is beyond imagination.

I am grateful to Dr. Cameron, my neurologist, who provided much hope and encouragement when I needed it the most. Each time I see you, I learn so much from you about life. Thank you for sharing your experiences and also providing a space for me to share mine. Meeting you has been one of the most amazing experiences of my life.

I would also like to express my gratitude to my physician, Dr. Davison, who knew about the level of brain tumor treatments in Los Angeles and encouraged me to follow the opportunity that had come my way. Thank you for your openness and for your utmost care. I am most fortunate to have you as my physician.

My heartfelt thanks also goes to my friend and former colleague, Barb Callander, who edited my initial manuscript. Your kindness and care as well as attention to detail is truly remarkable.

I am also very grateful to my family, particularly my sisters (Sheila, Mina, Lila, and Roya) and my brother-in-laws (Mehdi, Mohammad, and Farid) for being there with me on this journey from the start. There are no words to describe how much your love means to me.

I also would like to thank all my friends and students both in yoga and music who were a part of my journey. Thank you so much for your cards, phone calls, and words of encouragement. I have learned so much from all of you, and you inspire me to continue to learn and explore new ideas as a teacher.

And last, but by no means least, this book would not have been possible without the help of my special brother-in-law, Mehdi, who encouraged me and read my pages every week and called me to discuss them. Thanks so much for your tender response to my writing and for your encouragement to finish the book. Our phone conversations (which were sometimes more than two hours!) would themselves comprise an interesting book! Thank you with all my heart.

www.ingramcontent.com/pod-product-compliance
Lightning Source LLC
Chambersburg PA
CBHW052220270326
41931CB00011B/2420